RUN
SMART

NOTE

While every effort has been made to ensure that the content of this book is as technically accurate and as sound as possible, neither the author nor the publishers can accept responsibility for any injury or loss sustained as a result of the use of this material.

BLOOMSBURY SPORT
An imprint of Bloomsbury Publishing Plc

50 Bedford Square
London
WC1B 3DP
UK

1385 Broadway
New York
NY 10018
USA

www.bloomsbury.com

BLOOMSBURY and the Diana logo are trademarks of Bloomsbury Publishing Plc

First published 2017

© John Brewer, 2017

John Brewer has asserted his right under the Copyright, Designs and Patents Act, 1988, to be identified as Authors of this work.

British Library Cataloguing-in-Publication Data

A catalogue record for this book is available from the British Library.

ISBN PB: 9781472939685
ePDF: 9781472939708
ePub: 9781472939692

10 9 8 7 6 5 4 3 2 1

Inside photographs © Getty Images with the exception of the following; pp. 6 and 186 © MarathonFoto

Illustrations by Dave Gardner
Typeset in Minion Pro by bookdesigner.co.uk

Printed and bound in China by Toppan Leefung Printing Co

Bloomsbury Publishing Plc makes every effort to ensure that the papers used in the manufacture of our books are natural, recyclable products made from wood grown in well-managed forests. Our manufacturing processes conform to the environmental regulations of the country of origin.

To find out more about our authors and books visit **www.bloomsbury.com**. Here you will find extracts, author interviews, details of forthcoming events and the option to sign up for our newsletters.

All suggestions and material in this book are for information purposes only. Since each individual's personal situation, health history and lifestyle differs you should use discretion before proceeding to do any of the exercises or techniques described. The author and publisher expressly disclaim any responsibility for any adverse reactions or effects that may result from the use or interpretation of the information contained within this book.

RUN SMART

Using Science to Improve Performance and Expose Marathon Running's Greatest Myths

JOHN BREWER

BLOOMSBURY

LONDON · OXFORD · NEW YORK · NEW DELHI · SYDNEY

CONTENTS

Foreword by Greg James 6
Introduction 8

SECTION ONE

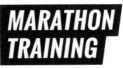

THE SCIENCE OF MARATHON RUNNING

A Scientific Approach to
  Marathon Training 12
Marathons – The Challenge to
  Metabolism 14
What Happens to Your Body When
  You Run a Marathon – a Mile-by
  -mile Breakdown 16
Running Speed – Getting the
  Intensity Right 20
The Science of Warming Up
  – Getting Ready for Action 22
Heart Rate, Oxygen Uptake and
  Body Temperature 24
Strides and Impact Forces 26
Pacing and Marathon-running Intensity
  – How High is Too High? 28
The Marathon and Our Vital Organs 32
Marathon Psychology 34
Marathon Nutrition 36
Marathon Hydration 38
Sleep 40
The Perfect Running Style 42
The Science of Race Tactics and
  Strategies 44
The Science of Running Kit 48
The Science of Older Running 50
The Science of Male and Female
  Runners 54
Striving to Improve 58
The Science of Speed Work 60
Survival Science 64
Breathing 66
Running Technology 68
Running at Altitude 70
The Science of Recovery 72
Thermoregulation – or Overheating 74
The Body Clock 76

SECTION TWO

MARATHON TRAINING

Starting Out 80
Training Principles 82
Assessing Your Fitness and Running
  Style 86
Different Training Approaches 88
Coaching and Running with Others 90
Setting an Achievable Target Time 92
Designing a Training Programme 96
Training Zones and Heart Rate
  Monitors 98
Training Nutrition 100
Training Hydration 102
Warming Up and Warming Down 104
Running in Different Weather
  Conditions 106
Cross-training 108
Injury Prevention and Listening
  to Your Body 110
Goal Setting 114
Coping With Illness 116
Overtraining 118
The Final Weeks and Tapering 122

SECTION THREE

RACE PREPARATION AND RACE DAY

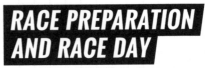

Pre-race Planning 128
Watch Out for the Weather 130
The Last Few Hours 132
Race-day Psychology 134
Race-day Nutrition 136
Race-day Hydration 138
Coping With Race Day 140
Race-day Strategy 144

SECTION FOUR

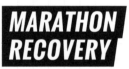

MARATHON RECOVERY

When the Marathon
is Over 150
Practical Steps for
Recovery 152

SECTION FIVE

NEW CHALLENGES

What Next? 156
The Marathon Majors 158
Marathons Made For
Scientists 160
Ultra-marathons 162

SECTION SIX

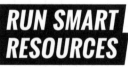

RUN SMART RESOURCES

100 Ways to Go 1 Per
Cent Faster 168
Basic Training
Programme 176
Advanced Training
Programme 178
Training Calendar 180
A Brief History of the
Marathon 182
Some Useful Tables 184

MARATHON MYTHS

- Not Everyone Can Run a Marathon 18
- Training is All About Long, Slow
  Running 18
- It's Not OK to be Overtaken 31
- Training for a Marathon Takes
  Over Your Life 31
- Marathon Running is All in the Mind 45
- Smaller Runners are Faster 47
- Marathon Runners Age Quicker 53
- You Need a Perfect Running Style 53
- Females Cope Better Than Males
  in Marathons 55
- It Takes Six Months to Train for
  a Marathon 57
- You Must Train for Five or Six
  Days Each Week 61
- You Need to Run 40–50 Miles
  Per Week 62
- Marathon Training is Boring 83
- If I Get Injured or ill I Will Have
  to Withdraw From My Marathon 85
- If I Can Run 20 miles, I Can Run
  a Marathon 95

- If I Run a Marathon I Will Lose
  Lots of Weight 95
- Marathon Running is Bad For You 111
- Heart Rate Monitors Are Essential 113
- You Should Not Run More Than Two
  or Three Marathons a Year 121
- Lactic Acid Causes Post-race
  Soreness 121
- Alcohol is Banned 125
- Eat as Many Carbs as Possible
  Before Race Day 125
- You Must Use Carbo Gels 142
- I Need a Good Start to Get a
  Good Time 143
- Nasal Strips Will Help Me to Breathe 145
- A Stitch Means Stopping 146
- You Can't Walk and Manage a
  Good Marathon Time 147
- Faster Running Burns More
  Calories Than Slow Running 147
- Taking Salt Cures Cramp 163
- You've Run out of Energy When you
  Hit the Wall 165

About the Author 186 / Index 188 / Acknowledgements 192

Greg James and John Brewer in high spirits as they complete the London Marathon together in 2015.

FOREWORD

Although I have done some half-marathons, the odd triathlon and a couple of full marathons, this stuff doesn't come naturally to me and I'd be lying if I said running 26.2 miles is something I would describe as a pleasure. But it can be done. Clearly. However, you must be prepared both physically and mentally. Marathons are tough, and that's what makes completing one, no matter what your time, such a tremendous achievement.

As hard as running a marathon can be, help is at hand in the form of Professor John Brewer, who not only understands the science of pounding the pavement, but has also personally completed 19 marathons. This research- and experience-based knowledge places John in a unique position to tell us the best way to take on the challenge as well as inform us of the many myths associated with marathon training. His words of wisdom will give you all you need to know to get you ready and keep you calm, and where to go in your mind when you're on mile 23 and you just can't be bothered any more. The latter is something that happened to me – and luckily, John was there!

Whether you are looking to shave seconds off your sub-3-hour time or just get around the course, *Run Smart* is packed with easy-to-understand, expert advice to help you to achieve your personal marathon-running objectives, and, dare I say it, make those 26.2 miles nearly a pleasure. It certainly helped me.

GREG JAMES

Finishing a marathon is the culmination of many weeks of hard work, determination and physical effort, but can be one of life's greatest experiences.

INTRODUCTION

Reading this book will not make running a marathon easy – but it may help to make it easier. The huge physical and mental challenges of training and completing the 26.2-mile distance cannot and must not be underestimated. This book provides a comprehensive overview of the many different areas that it is essential to get right if a marathon is to be accomplished successfully, and demonstrates how advances in science can be applied to all aspects of marathon preparation and competition. The book is aimed at runners of all abilities – whether you are a nervous novice aiming to complete the distance, or a serious veteran hoping to shave just a few seconds off your personal best time. Throughout each section, the book also seeks to explode many myths that surround marathon running, and show that while completing a marathon will always be a huge accomplishment, the correct application of a science-based approach to training, preparing for, and running a marathon makes the 26.2 miles a more manageable and successful experience.

Within the six sections of this book, the parallel paths of the growth in marathon running, and the advancement of marathon science, are brought together in an easy-to-understand and informative way that will motivate and support any runner during their quest to complete a marathon. The application of science to all aspects of marathon training – preparation, planning, performance and recovery – is a common theme throughout each section. Regardless of experience or personal-best time, the book contains science-based advice that will be of some benefit to novices and more experienced marathon runners alike. Section One explores the science of marathon running, and the stresses that are placed on the human body as it copes with and adapts to the experience. In Section Two, the science behind training is explored in greater detail, along with how best to apply this to properly prepare for a marathon. This section also shows how runners can cope and adapt to the inevitable challenges of injury and illness, and how to deal with the crucial final few days before the race itself. Section Three focuses on race day, and how to use science to manage critical areas such as nutrition, hydration, nerves and pacing, as well as explaining the best methods for coping with a crisis if things do happen to go wrong. Section Four covers the optimal way to recover once the race has been completed, with top tips on how to return to normal post-marathon life. Section Five highlights potential new challenges and possible alternative marathons, while Section Six provides examples of practical training programmes that could be used to further enhance the experience of marathon running. Each section also includes a series of marathon myths that are debunked with science, thus dispelling many of the barriers and false assumptions around marathons and running that have developed over many years.

Reading this book will not guarantee marathon success. That requires many miles of training, combined with physical and mental resilience. But not reading this book, and failing to apply the sound scientific principles behind marathon training and running that are contained within it, will almost certainly make your marathon-running experience much harder. Using the advice in *Run Smart*, Chris Brasher's 'suburban man's Everest' will become a lot easier to climb!

Marathon Running is an immense challenge, but applying science to training and racing can make marathons much easier.

THE SCIENCE OF MARATHON RUNNING

During the course of a marathon, immense stresses will be placed on the body. Sports science not only measures this, but can also be used to help your body cope and work in the most efficient manner possible.

A SCIENTIFIC APPROACH TO MARATHON TRAINING

From Ancient Greece to the modern Olympics, and in towns and cities around the world, marathons have become a pinnacle of achievement for many endurance runners.

The human body is designed to run – our ancient ancestors had to run to catch food, or run slightly faster to avoid being food for a predator. Whether or not we are designed to run 26.2 miles is another matter though. Scientists have shown that the two biggest challenges faced by runners during a marathon are the relentless emptying of the body's stores of fuel and fluid, and there are many other factors which combine to create the physical and mental fatigue that make finishing the distance such an achievement.

When Pheidippides completed the first marathon in 490 BC, sports science did not exist. Had it done so, it is possible that the advice he would have had access to in advance of his run from Sparta to Athens would have prevented him from dropping dead when he finished. Today, our knowledge of sport and exercise science, and sports nutrition, has advanced to the extent that it now plays a fundamental part in the training, preparation, completion and recovery from a marathon. Although the application of scientific knowledge will never make a marathon easy, choosing to ignore the advice and insight that science now brings to marathon running greatly increases the chances of at worst, failure, or at best, a poor performance.

Understanding the science of marathon training and running can help to make the vital differences that separate a great race that will live long in the memory, from a terrible one that no runner will ever wish to repeat. For example, appreciating the importance of transporting oxygen from air that enters the lungs to the muscles that provide energy is critical in the design of a marathon-training programme. Without understanding the vital role played by the body's limited stores of carbohydrate in the provision of fuel, it is all too easy to get race-day nutritional strategies wrong. Today, our knowledge of the science of hydration – particularly in hot and humid conditions – can make the difference between effectively maintaining core temperature, or dehydrating and overheating during the run.

Scientists have studied and understood the role of mental preparation and 'mind strategies' when tackling endurance

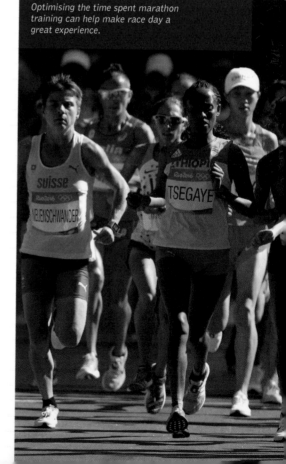

Optimising the time spent marathon training can help make race day a great experience.

events such as marathons. Overcoming the inevitable mental demons that can overwhelm runners and exacerbate fatigue is crucial for marathon success, since they pose as great a challenge as the physical aspects of going the distance.

Marathon training and running places huge stresses on the body, and inevitably there is a risk of injury and illness. However, advances in science have shown how these risks can be minimised through sensible selection of clothing and footwear, correct training, and exercises to develop strength and mobility.

On race day, sticking to sensible, science-based practices from waking up until crossing the finishing line will help to ensure success. These include understanding the scientific basis of pacing during the marathon – scientists have shown that elite runners complete the course at a high proportion of their maximum capacity, while recreational runners run at a lower capacity.

However, if recreational runners set off too quickly – and run at a proportion of their maximum capacity that is too high – it has been demonstrated that, while they might feel great for the first few miles, physiological 'damage' starts immediately, with energy and fluid stores depleting quickly, and body temperature rapidly rising.

Science can also support the post-race recovery process. Nutritional scientists have identified the optimum foods and drinks for recovery, and how to time their post-race intake. While most runners will not want to run – or be capable of running – for a few days after a marathon, using science to enhance recovery will go a long way towards preparing them for their next challenge. In the following section, we will explore the demands placed on a runner's body as a marathon unfolds, and show how these accumulate to produce fatigue towards the end of the race – a feeling that experienced marathon runners will know only too well!

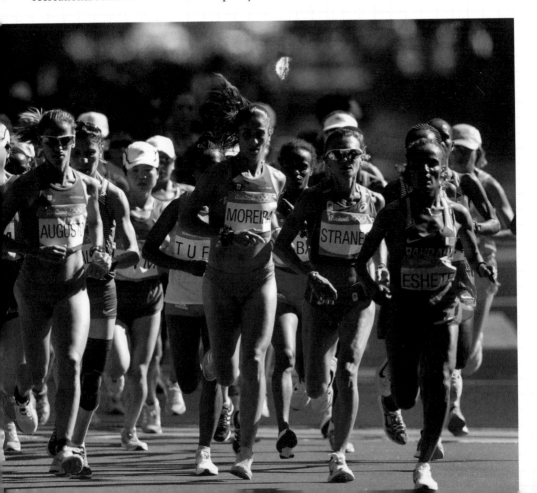

MARATHONS – THE CHALLENGE TO METABOLISM

Requiring large amounts of energy, and elevating the metabolism to levels far higher than those found at rest, coping with the metabolic demands of marathons is the greatest test faced by runners.

Why are marathons tough? The simple reason is that running 26.2 miles places physical demands on the human body that are way above those experienced during our normal daily lives. Completing the 35,000 strides that carry most runners from the start to the finish represents a challenge that takes the body to the very limits of human endurance.

When we start to run a marathon, the body's requirement for energy quickly increases four-fold from that required at rest. There is an immediate rise in heart rate and breathing frequency so that more blood and oxygen can be supplied to the muscles. By the time the finish line is reached, the heart will have made around 40,000 beats and approximately 25,000 litres (44,000 pints) of air will have travelled in and out of a runner's lungs. Body temperature will be rising steadily, and could soon reach boiling point unless heat is lost. Sweating is the runner's first line of defence against this build-up of heat, and in hot and humid conditions sweat can evaporate from the skin at rates of 1–2 litres (1¾–3½ pints) an hour. By

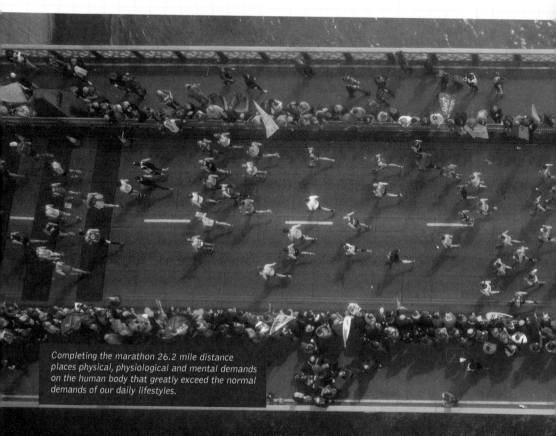

Completing the marathon 26.2 mile distance places physical, physiological and mental demands on the human body that greatly exceed the normal demands of our daily lifestyles.

understanding the demands that marathons place on the body, we can optimise training programmes and preparation strategies to ensure that runners either improve or, if they are first-timers, have the best possible experience when completing the distance.

At rest, most of us burn about 3 calories per minute. However, as soon as running starts, this can easily increase to 10–15 calories per minute (the exact amount will depend on running speed, efficiency and body size). Factor in the need to continue this rate of energy expenditure for the time it takes to cover 26.2 miles, and it is easy to see why runners often experience such high rates of fatigue during the latter stages of a marathon.

Do faster marathon runners use more energy than slower ones? The simple answer is 'no'. Although the rate at which faster runners generate energy is higher than that of slower ones, the total energy required to cover a mile, or indeed 26.2 miles, is pretty much the same for all runners regardless of speed. The main determinant of total energy expenditure is bodyweight and running efficiency, since the laws of physics dictate that more energy is needed to move a heavier mass than is needed to move a lighter mass, provided the distance is the same.

Most runners use around 120 calories when covering each mile, which come from the body's stores of fat and carbohydrate. Each gram of fat contains around 9 calories of energy and, as a result, we have enough stored 'fat calories' to fuel approximately 40 consecutive marathons! Conversely, the stores of carbohydrate – known as glycogen – only amount to around 2000–2500 calories, or enough for 18–20 miles of running. This presents us with a potential energy crisis, since carbohydrate is the body's preferred fuel for all but the slowest running speeds. For runners of all abilities, the main challenge is to run at a pace that uses energy in the most efficient way, finishing the marathon as safely and quickly as possible, but without exhausting the supply of energy.

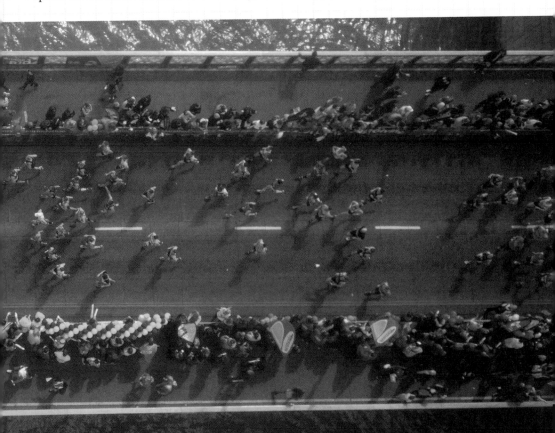

WHAT HAPPENS TO YOUR BODY WHEN YOU RUN A MARATHON – A MILE-BY-MILE BREAKDOWN

Marathons place ever-increasing stresses on the human body. This section highlights the mile-by-mile effects, and how these lead to physical and mental exhaustion.

Marathon runners accumulate fatigue as each completed mile slowly saps the body of energy and fluid. An awareness of how marathon fatigue develops is an important first step in fully appreciating the demands of the event, and in the design of strategies that help runners to cope more effectively.

START TO MILE 4

■ At the start, you should be feeling nervous, but in great shape. When the starting gun goes, your muscles need more energy, so within the mitochondria – the powerhouse of the muscle – a complex biochemical process called the Krebs cycle produces energy-rich adenosine triphosphate (ATP). Carbohydrate stores (glycogen) support this process, along with some contribution from fat.

■ Your heart rate will quickly increase to approximately 150 beats per minute, and core temperature will start to rise due to a build-up of heat that is a by-product of energy production.

■ Breathing frequency and oxygen uptake will increase and plateau, and adrenalin levels – which will be high on the start line – start to drop.

■ The body will enter a physiological 'steady state' during the first 4 miles, and the changes from resting levels at the start will have stabilised, ready for the challenge ahead.

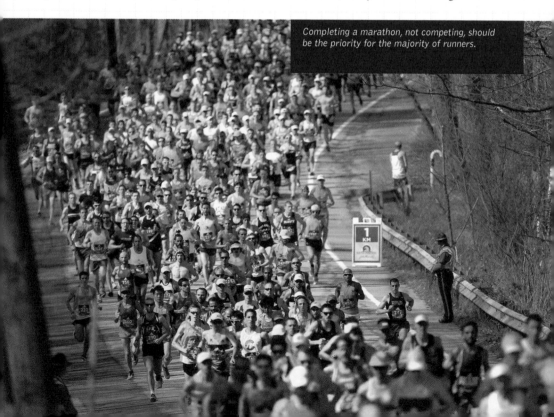

Completing a marathon, not competing, should be the priority for the majority of runners.

MILES 4–8

- Relaxation is key at this stage – conserving energy, feeling good and staying positive are essential.
- The physiological steady state will continue with no dramatic changes, and after its initial rise, core temperature will plateau at around 2°C (3.5°F) higher than it was at rest.
- Glands secrete sweat on to the surface of the skin, and latent heat is lost through evaporation.
- Blood flow to the skin's surface increases, aiding heat loss as warm blood loses heat to the external environment.
- There will be some early signs of dehydration, with the potential for around 2 litres (3½ pints) of fluid to have been lost by this stage.

MILES 8–13

- By this stage, you will be experiencing the first effects of fatigue. Stores of carbohydrate (glycogen) will show signs of depletion, and over 1000 calories have now been used.
- Sweating continues to deplete fluid stores unless on-course drinks are used, but there should be no significant rise in core temperature.
- Lactic acid – a main cause of fatigue during intensive exercise – will have increased slightly, but should not be high enough to impact on running performance.
- Heart rate and oxygen uptake remain constant.

13.1 MILES: HALFWAY

- A significant psychological milestone – depending on the effort needed to reach halfway, this will either be a landmark that results in a 'can do' attitude for the remaining distance, or it will produce negative thoughts that make the remaining challenge even harder.

MILES 13.1–17

- This is a crucial stage of the race, when aches and pains will become apparent.
- Glycogen stores will have decreased substantially, and the body will start drawing on its reserves of fat, which requires more oxygen to produce energy, so the effort needed to sustain a constant pace will increase.
- The relentless impact on the ground and continual use of muscles, tendons and ligaments will be starting to cause aches, pains and abrasions.

MILES 17–21

- Psychologically, a difficult time, and negative thoughts could combine with fatigue to reduce running pace.
- Energy expenditure will have reached and possibly exceeded 2000 calories, and fluid loss may be in excess of 4 litres (7 pints).
- Glycogen stores are low and the body is increasingly reliant on fat for energy.

MILES 21–26

- Dehydration will be a major challenge, with fluid loss exceeding 2 per cent of body weight.
- Sweating will have caused a loss of crucial electrolytes, such as sodium and potassium, impairing muscle and nerve function, and increasing the risk of cramp.
- Glycogen stores will be almost fully depleted and running style may change to relieve tired muscles, and to tap into any remaining glycogen in other muscle fibres.
- Core temperature may start to rise again as additional effort is needed to continue running.

26.2 MILES

- As you cross the finish line, glycogen stores will be completely depleted, you will be dehydrated and may have lost around 6 litres (10½ pints) of sweat.
- There will be sores, blisters, and damage to muscle fibres due to overuse, persistent rubbing, and impact with the ground.
- Despite all this, the feeling of euphoria from finishing will produce endorphins that mask pain, creating a (temporary) 'high' now that 26.2 miles has been completed.

In conclusion, a marathon sustains demands on the body that push it to its limits of endurance, but by understanding these demands, and their scientific basis, we can start to develop strategies to overcome them.

MYTH: *NOT EVERYONE CAN RUN A MARATHON*

There was a time when only males were allowed to compete in marathons, and anyone finishing in anything more than 3 hours could well have found that by the time they reached the finish line, everyone else had left and gone home.

Today, however, marathons have become mass-participation events that are open to men and women, from 18 years of age to 100 years of age, and the cut-off time for completing the distance extends to many hours. Marathons remain an extreme physical and mental challenge, and while running one in a fast time remains an achievable goal for many, completing one at a steady yet realistic pace is an attainable goal for many more.

Take the London Marathon for example. Finishers must complete the distance in less than 8 hours if they are to receive a medal and official time. That's equivalent to an average speed of 3.3 miles per hour, or around 18 minutes for each mile – about the same speed as a steady walk. However, given that we are all designed to run at a pace that is much faster than this, and our bodies are all capable of adapting to the stimulus of regular training, it is certainly possible for the vast majority of people to train and successfully complete a marathon in a respectable time – so long as their goals are realistic, they follow a sensible training programme and lifestyle, and have realistic targets when the day of the race arrives.

MYTH: *TRAINING IS ALL ABOUT LONG, SLOW RUNNING*

Training changes the body's physiology. This is because it will experience an intensity of exercise and overload that is greater than that to which it is exposed in everyday life. Some coaches used to advocate a policy of 'no pain, no gain' – in other words if training were not hard and painful, it would not have any benefit. However, sports scientists have shown that this is not the case, and that lower-intensity training also has benefits.

Marathon runners need to be able to spend a long time on their feet running, so long, slow running is always going to play an important part in the training programme for any marathon. However, runners also need to incorporate higher-intensity training into their programmes, since the higher

overload from these sessions will develop maximum capacity, and consequently make the long, slow runs much easier. Simply running long distances slowly will train the body to do one thing well – run long distances slowly. By including shorter, high-intensity training, variable pace running, and speed and hill work, runners will add variety to a marathon-training programme. This will develop their capacity to cope with higher-intensity, faster speeds, while making lower-intensity, slower speeds – the sort that are likely to be sustained for a marathon – feel much easier.

Adding high-intensity training to a programme that also contains long, slow distance work will therefore result in optimal training programmes and well-trained marathon runners.

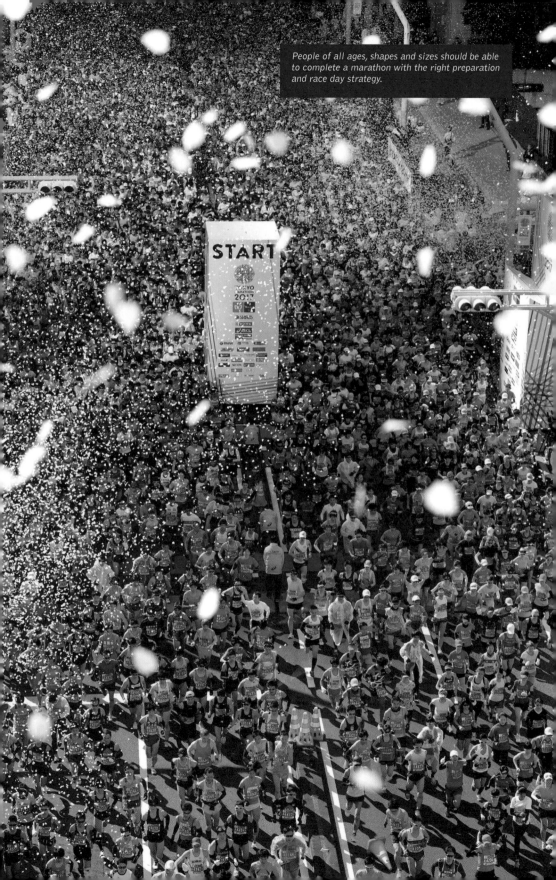

People of all ages, shapes and sizes should be able to complete a marathon with the right preparation and race day strategy.

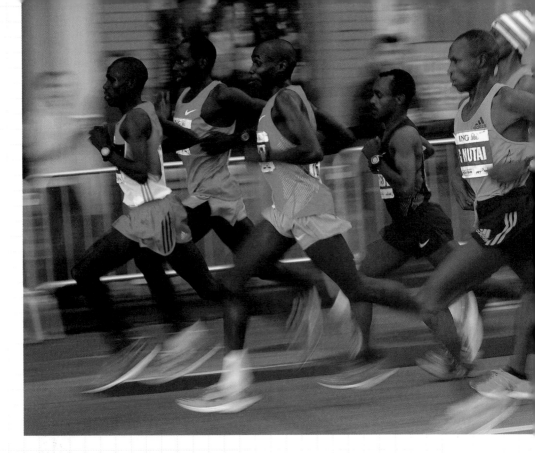

RUNNING SPEED – GETTING THE INTENSITY RIGHT

Our physiological systems react to the intensity of a run – too high, and things go wrong; too low, and the run takes longer. Getting the intensity right is a crucial component of marathon success.

At the same constant pace, all runners experience different levels of fatigue. I once ran with Olympic 1500m champion Sebastian Coe – he was smiling and relaxed, since relative to his normal pace he was running at a much lower intensity, whereas I was going all out. This difference in experience is important, since a runner's exercise intensity during a marathon has a significant impact on the body's ability to cope with the distance.

If a group of runners set off at the same pace, they will immediately increase the supply of oxygen to their muscles to support energy production. Scientists normally refer to this oxygen supply as 'VO2', an abbreviation for 'volume of oxygen'. Larger, heavier runners will need a higher VO2 than smaller runners, due to their greater body mass, but when VO2 is 'normalised' to take bodyweight into account, the value will be very similar for the entire group. In this context, VO2 is expressed in millilitres of oxygen per kilogram of bodyweight (ml/kg/min). Laboratory experiments have found that on average, runners use around 5ml/

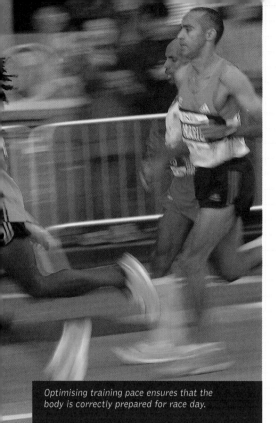
Optimising training pace ensures that the body is correctly prepared for race day.

max of 50ml/kg/min will find things slightly easier, since they will be close to 80 per cent of maximum capacity, while if there was a highly trained elite runner in the group, with a VO2 max of 80ml/kg/min, they would only be running at 50 per cent of maximum capacity, and finding the pace very easy.

This percentage of maximum running speed is known as a runner's 'relative exercise intensity' or REI. The REI has crucial implications for an individual's response to exercise, and is far more relevant than the actual running speed. Many other physiological variables are closely related to the REI – these include heart rate, core temperature, the metabolism of energy stores, and the distribution of blood flow to the stomach and gut. The lower a runner's REI, the less likely they are to experience fatigue, and they will use more fat as an energy store rather than carbohydrate, something that is vital during the early stages of a marathon.

Scientists have found that elite highly trained runners can sustain an REI of close to 80 per cent during the race, whereas recreational runners can only sustain an REI of 70 per cent. Interestingly, this ability to sustain an REI may be related to time rather than distance – elite runners generally complete the 26.2-mile marathon distance in 2–2½ hours, whereas the times of recreational runners can easily be twice as long. It is unlikely that elite runners would be able to sustain a pace of 80 per cent of maximum for 4 or 5 hours, but they are fortunate that a combination of their high VO2 max and training means that their pace at 80 per cent REI enables them to complete the distance quickly. Runners with a lower VO2 max who try to sustain a high REI will simply not be running fast enough to finish the distance before they fatigue, and as a result they are forced to run at a lower percentage of their maximum capacity.

So, running at the right intensity – one that suits you and not those around you – is critical for successful completion of 26.2 miles. Since the physiological responses of the body are closely linked to running intensity, getting it wrong can have disastrous consequences.

kg/min of oxygen for each mile per hour of running speed. So, if our group were running each mile in a time of 7 minutes 30 seconds, equivalent to a speed of 8 miles per hour, most would have a VO2 of 8 x 5ml, or approximately 40ml/kg/min.

However, closer examination of this group would soon show that despite the similar oxygen cost of running, some will be finding it far harder than others. The reason for this is quite simple – it will depend on what fraction of their maximum capacity that 40ml/kg/min represents. This maximum capacity – more commonly known as VO2 max – represents the maximum amount of oxygen that the body can utilise per minute, and is widely recognised by scientists, coaches and athletes as one of the best determinants of endurance-running performance. To explain further, if a runner in our group has a VO2 max of 40ml/kg/min, they will find that a pace of 7 minutes 30 seconds per mile is close to 100 per cent of maximum capacity. A runner with a VO2

THE SCIENCE OF WARMING UP – GETTING READY FOR ACTION

Is warming up necessary for marathons, and how long should it take? Getting the balance right between preparing properly while not expending too much energy is part of the secret of marathon success.

In this section, we will explore the scientific basis of warming up for a marathon, alongside the potential risks if we get the warm-up wrong. We start by reviewing the process that creates movement, which helps to understand what a warm-up should focus on. As well as exploring the scientific justification for warming up, we will also explore the benefits of warming down when a run has been completed.

The muscles that produce energy for running are known as skeletal muscles, consisting of microscopic fibres, which in turn contain many millions of protein filaments that are drawn together to shorten the muscle and move the limbs. When muscles shorten, they kick-start a chain of forces and movements involving tendons, ligaments, bones and joints, all coordinated by nerve impulses, that propel and stabilise the running body.

> **'Failure to warm up means that energy is produced less efficiently, movement is harder due to lack of muscle, tendon and ligament elasticity and, as a consequence, the risk of injury is increased.'**

The biochemical process contracting the muscle filaments and fibres is complex, involving enzymes, reactions, and the breakdown of adenosine triphosphate (ATP) to release energy. As with any chemical reaction, this process occurs more efficiently and rapidly in a warm environment. The contraction forces create movement within the muscles, tendons and ligaments, often rapidly and through a large range of movement and, again, this happens more efficiently, and with less risk of injury, within a warm environment; like any material, these structures are brittle when cold, but more pliable and elastic when warm.

The energy-producing process is supported by the supply of oxygen to the muscles, carried by haemoglobin in the blood, which is pumped around the body by the heart. Unless the heart responds quickly to the demand for extra energy and increases blood flow, there will soon be an 'oxygen debt' as the rate of energy that is needed exceeds the rate at which oxygen can be supplied to muscles.

The secret to preparing the body for exercise and creating the optimum pre-run physiological environment for exercise is what is commonly referred to as 'warming up'. This pre-race or pre-training run period is the time when runners need to elevate core and muscle temperature before exercise starts, so that the internal environment within the body is optimised for the efficient production of energy. Failure to warm up means that energy is produced less efficiently, movement is harder due to lack of muscle, tendon and ligament elasticity and, as a consequence, the risk of injury is increased. Warming up also starts to elevate the heart rate, cardiac output and blood flow to the muscles, ensuring that the body is prepared for the more rigorous exercise that is about to follow. There are psychological benefits from warming up too – it is a time when runners can focus on the mental challenge ahead, cutting out external 'noise' to concentrate on the tactics and strategy that they will soon need to employ.

Once the warm-up has been completed, the body is ready for action and as prepared as it can be for the many thousands of strides

'A more gradual return to normal, controlled by light exercise once the run is over, may help to enhance recovery and reduce post-exercise muscle soreness.'

that will be taken once the gun goes.

During a run, the body's metabolism increases to a higher level, with many physiological variables such as heart rate, core temperature and oxygen uptake being significantly higher than they are at rest. Depending on the intensity of the run, there may also be an increase in lactic acid levels and consequently an increase in the acidity of the blood. While it is always tempting to stop suddenly at the end of a training session and of course at the end of a marathon, this is not advisable. Instead, you should warm down – a technique used to gradually reduce these measures to normal. Stopping quickly can lead to a sudden decrease in blood flow to areas such as the brain, and a 'pooling' of lactic acid in the muscles occurs if heart rate and blood flow drop rapidly. A more gradual return to normal, controlled by light exercise once the run is over, may help to enhance recovery and reduce post-exercise muscle soreness.

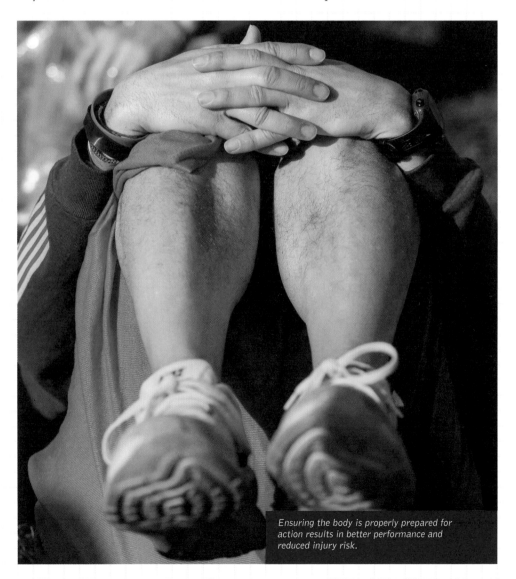

Ensuring the body is properly prepared for action results in better performance and reduced injury risk.

HEART RATE, OXYGEN UPTAKE AND BODY TEMPERATURE

When a marathon starts, the body reacts to the demand for extra energy. Coping with this demand places physiological stresses on the body that have to be sustained for 26.2 miles.

Standing on the start line, most runners' hearts will be beating at a rate of between 60 and 70 beats per minute, and using around 3ml of oxygen for each 1kg (2.2lb) of bodyweight. At the same time, body temperature will be at its resting level of around 37°C (99°F). However, as soon as the starting gun sounds, all of this will change as the body moves from a state of rest to one of action.

Running requires energy, and in human beings, releasing energy requires oxygen. There is plenty of it around – about one-fifth of our atmosphere is oxygen – but getting it to the muscles quickly and efficiently is a challenge. The first stage in this process is to draw more air into the lungs by breathing more deeply and frequently. This enables oxygen to transfer across the membranes of the lungs, into the bloodstream, where it attaches to a substance in the blood called haemoglobin.

'...scientific studies have found that in marathon runners [the heart rate] can soon rise to around 150 beats per minute.'

Normally, at rest, the heart will pump around 5 litres (8¾ pints) of blood around the body each minute. If this remains the same when running commences, it will not be possible to meet the muscles' increased demand for oxygen, and running will soon cease. So, the body reacts by increasing its heart rate from its resting level, and scientific studies have found that in marathon runners this can soon rise to around 150 beats per minute, increasing the volume of blood pumped around the body to around 30 litres (52¾ pints) per minute. When the marathon

runners' oxygen-saturated haemoglobin reaches the contracting muscles, it lets go of the oxygen, which then enters the muscle cell where it is quickly used to support the production of energy. Blood that still contains haemoglobin, but now with less oxygen, returns to the heart and lungs to collect more oxygen, before returning again to the muscles, so that energy can continually be

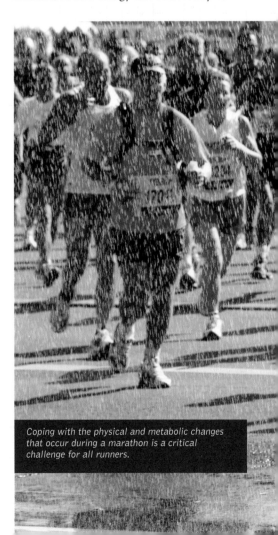

Coping with the physical and metabolic changes that occur during a marathon is a critical challenge for all runners.

produced for each stride of the marathon. From an oxygen uptake of just 3ml/kg/min at rest, values of 30–60ml/kg/min can quickly and easily be reached, depending on a runner's fitness and speed.

When muscles produce energy, they also produce heat, and this heat needs to be lost if the body is not going to overheat. From around 37°C (99°F) at rest, body temperature – or core temperature – will quickly and inexorably start to rise as the marathon progresses.

Some of this heat is lost through the air that is breathed out, but very quickly the temperature of the blood, muscles, tissues and internal organs will start to rise. At first this is not an issue, since a warm muscle is a more efficient one, and is also more pliable and less prone to injury. However, in order to prevent a dangerous build-up of heat, there needs to be an efficient heat-loss process, and the evaporation of sweat from the skin is the body's main mechanism for doing this. As a result, sweating starts not long into the race, and it is important that runners do all they can – particularly by wearing appropriate running clothing – to allow sweat to evaporate effectively. Sweat absorbed by clothing, or that drips from the body, is not as efficient at losing heat when compared with sweat that is allowed to evaporate.

Once the rate of heat loss matches the rate of heat production, core temperature will plateau, as will heart rate, oxygen uptake and breathing frequency. The body will have reached a 'steady state' that should feel comfortable and tolerable, and every marathon runner's challenge should now be to sustain this until the finish line is reached.

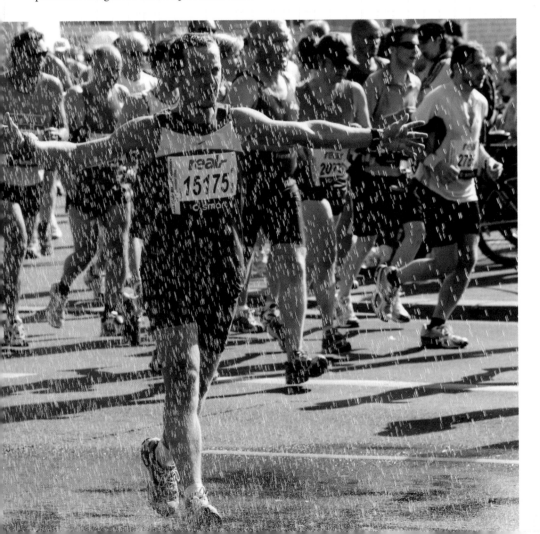

STRIDES AND IMPACT FORCES

Marathons are all about taking lots of strides. Simply putting one foot in front of the other and creating the forces needed to propel the body is the essence of completing the 26.2-mile distance.

No two runners have an identical running style, but the basic principles of the running stride are the same regardless of age and ability. Some runners look ungainly, yet their style works and 'feels right' for them – others look as if they are effortlessly covering the ground at high speed. However, common to all runners is the impact of their feet on the ground, and the generation of force to move the runner forwards.

Completing a marathon requires a significant number of strides to get from the start to the finish line. The time that it takes to cover the distance is also a simple function of stride rate multiplied by stride frequency, since this determines running speed. For example, a runner with a stride length of 1.2m (3.8ft) and a stride rate of 170 strides per minute will be running at a pace of 204m per minute – which is 12.2km per hour or 7.6 miles per hour – and a final marathon time of 3 hours 27 minutes. In this scenario, the runner would be taking around 35,000 strides (or 17,500 strides with each leg) to complete the distance. Closer investigation of marathon running has shown that it is normal for runners to take this number of strides to cover the distance, with many taking far more when stride length shortens as a result of fatigue during the latter part of the race.

Each stride is produced by the complex interaction of muscles, tendons and ligaments within the hips and lower limbs and the impact

All the force needed to propel the body 26.2 miles comes from the feet hitting the ground when running or walking.

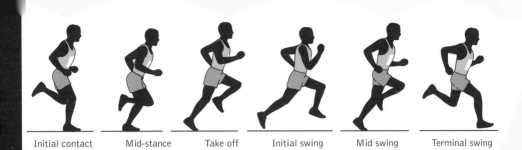

| Initial contact | Mid-stance | Take off | Initial swing | Mid swing | Terminal swing |

of the feet with the ground, which produce a propulsion force to move the body forwards.

The study of running strides is known as 'biomechanics', with each individual stride called the 'gait cycle'. When running, the gait cycle is distinctive since at no time are both feet in contact with the ground simultaneously, unlike when walking. The impact of the front foot with the ground produces the 'drive phase', after which the body's centre of gravity passes over this foot moving it to the rear until it lifts from the ground. The movement of the foot and limb back to the front of the body is known as the 'swing phase'.

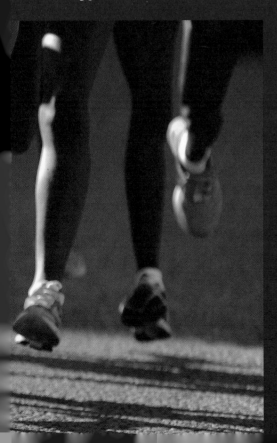

Although not everyone runs in the same way, scientists have shown that 80 per cent of runners make their drive phase impact with the rear of their foot, before rotating forwards from their mid-foot to the forefoot and toes until it lifts to commence the swing phase. Regardless of running speed, biomechanical analysis of runners has found that there is a short period of deceleration each time the foot impacts with the ground, and minimising this is an important determinant of running efficiency. Analysis of the impact of the foot with the ground has shown that a force of approximately two-and-a-half times the runner's bodyweight is produced. For a runner weighing 70kg (11st or 154lb), this is equivalent to a 175kg (27st 7lb, or 386lb) impact with each footfall, or over 3,000,000kg (472,420st, or 6,614,000lb) of total impact when multiplied 17,500 times for each leg.

Biomechanical analysis of running and runners' styles often results in attempts to change gait to improve efficiency and performance. However, subsequent studies suggest that the benefits of doing this may not be great, with most runners tending to subconsciously favour and use a running style that is best suited to their own anatomy and biomechanics, even if this appears ungainly and inefficient.

Strides, and lots of them, are what marathons are all about. All runners have different strides, and they change over the course of 26.2 miles. Getting your strides right, and dealing with their impact, is crucial for marathon success.

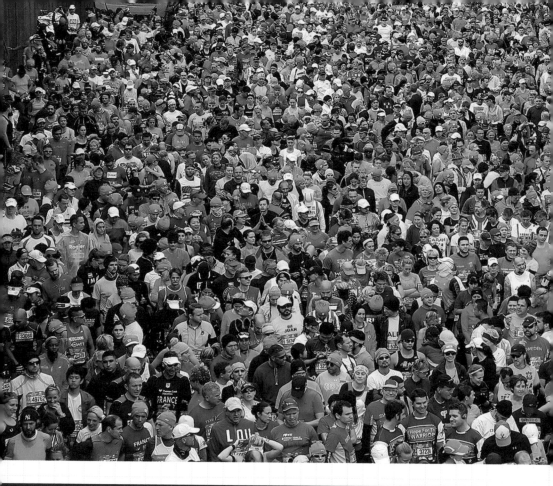

PACING AND MARATHON-RUNNING INTENSITY – HOW HIGH IS TOO HIGH?

The intensity at which marathons are run has a significant impact on the physiological strain placed on the body – knowing how hard to push is vital if fatigue is to be avoided.

You won't be alone if you are nervous at the start of a marathon – the majority of other runners will be feeling the same. The scientific cause of this feeling is the secretion of the hormone adrenalin, which prepares the body for action by increasing heart rate and dilating blood vessels, improving the supply of blood and oxygen to the muscles. This innate physiological reaction to impending exercise is known as the 'flight-or-fight' response, and when the

start gun goes, it is clearly a long 'flight' that is required!

The downside of the flight-or-fight response is that it can easily lead to an early pace that is too fast, often exacerbated by the pace of other runners, your competitive instinct, and in the case of large marathons, crowds of cheering spectators. Runners should feel good on the start line – your training will be over and your body will be prepared for action. But 26.2 miles is a long

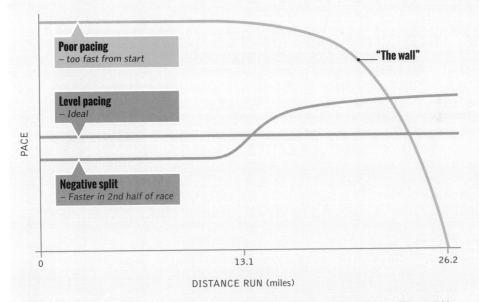

Excitement will be high at the start, but controlling this and starting at a sensible pace is essential.

Poor pacing
— too fast from start

"The wall"

Level pacing
— Ideal

Negative split
— Faster in 2nd half of race

PACE

0   13.1   26.2

DISTANCE RUN (miles)

A graph showing the difference between good and bad pacing, and the effect of setting off too quickly.

way, and the early pace needs to be one that feels as close to being effortless as possible. Setting off at anything more than a pace that feels more than light effort must be avoided, since one that is too fast immediately incurs physiological and metabolic damage beneath the skin and within the muscles.

The human body has two stores of energy that will fuel your marathon: fat and carbohydrate. Fat stores are abundant, whereas carbohydrate stores (glycogen) are limited to energy for just 18–20 miles of running. In an ideal world, the body would use fat to fuel a marathon, but unfortunately fat only provides energy at a slow rate, and requires a large amount of oxygen to do so. Conversely, the limited glycogen stores are more efficient, producing energy at a faster rate than fat, and use less oxygen to do so.

Stimulated by the flight-or-fight response, and the competitive excitement of the race, it is all too easy to set off at a pace that is quicker than planned. Since energy is needed rapidly, glycogen becomes the only source of fuel, and consequently the glycogen 'burn rate' is high. If this fast pace continues, glycogen stores will be depleted long before the finish line (a situation often referred to as 'hitting the wall'), and when this happens, fat becomes the only viable source of fuel. The high oxygen cost of acquiring energy from the metabolism of less-efficient fat immediately makes running feel much harder, and as a result, running pace almost inevitably drops. For many, this leads to a significantly slower latter part of the race, with walking commonplace.

The sensible alternative is to stick rigidly to a strategy of easy, slow pacing during the early and mid-stages of the race. This enables your body to obtain more energy from fat, saving the carbohydrate stores for the very end of the race. Although this means you will be moving more slowly over the early stages of the race, I have found that this is more than compensated for with a higher pace over the final miles.

Research I have conducted on the 2014 London Marathon found that, on average, runners slowed by 30 per cent during the second half of the race, yet much of this decrement could have been avoided with a slower, 'carb-sparing' pace at the start. Despite all the warnings, over half of the runners set off too quickly, and pay the price with fatigue at the end. Completing, not competing, should be the goal, especially for novices, and proper pacing is a crucial ingredient for marathon success.

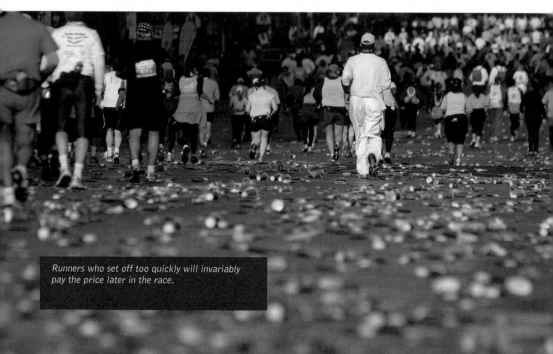

Runners who set off too quickly will invariably pay the price later in the race.

MYTH: *IT'S NOT OK TO BE OVERTAKEN*

There is a competitive streak in all of us, and no runner, no matter how fast or slow, likes to be overtaken. But running 26.2 miles really is a marathon and not a sprint, and being overtaken in the early stages of the race is – for the majority of runners – nothing to worry about – and in fact often an indication of sensible pacing. In most races, the majority of marathon runners set off too quickly, and pay the price towards the end. A smaller minority are sensible, starting slowly and running at a steady pace for the entire distance. This takes great self-control at the start, as runners of all shapes, sizes and ages speed past, looking good and appearing to run effortlessly. This is not a time to try to join them, since it is highly likely that they will be caught and passed later in the run. The temptation to speed up and stay with faster runners must be avoided, and this danger is at its greatest when the difference in running pace is quite small. For example, when a runner overtakes a fellow competitor who is running just 30 seconds per mile slower, the speed difference can appear negligible, and it is all too easy for the slower runner to accelerate to keep up. However, this can have disastrous consequences, as 30 seconds per mile equates to a difference of almost 15 minutes in final finishing time. Running your own race, at your own speed, and ignoring the pace of others around you, is crucial.

MYTH: *TRAINING FOR A MARATHON TAKES OVER YOUR LIFE*

Marathons are major events in the lives of both novice and experienced marathon runners, and most will rightly say that the hardest part of a marathon is the miles and hours of training and the consequent impact on lifestyle, rather than the race itself. There is no doubt that marathon training requires a significant amount of time and effort, but with sensible planning and the support of others close to you there is no need for it to totally dominate your life. The secret is to schedule running into set days and times during the week – times at which you have limited distractions, which are non-negotiable. For some, these could be early mornings, for others lunch times or evenings. Weekends are also key times when most runners are able to find the time for longer runs.

Training does not – in fact should not – need to be on every day of the week, since fitting in recovery time is more important than an extra run. For runners who are less worried about personal-best times and more concerned with completing the distance, marathons can be completed on three or four training sessions per week, provided that the programme is sensible and includes a weekly long run that gradually increases in distance as race day approaches.

Of course marathon training will change your life, but it does not need to completely dominate it. For many it can actually provide a welcome focus and distraction from the normal daily routine.

THE MARATHON AND OUR VITAL ORGANS

Our vital organs have to cope with the body's shifting priorities during marathon running, with blood flow changing to reflect the body's needs and the varying importance of each organ.

THE BRAIN

Our brains need fuel just like the rest of the body. Unlike our muscles, which use glycogen, the brain uses glucose for energy, which is supplied by the blood. Protecting the functioning of the brain is a high priority, so blood supply is maintained at all costs. However, as a marathon enters its latter stages and the point at which blood-glucose levels could start to drop, energy supply to the brain may be reduced, which can lead to light-headedness and confusion.

THE HEART

Probably the world's most efficient pump, running a marathon causes the heart to beat around 150 times per minute, or about 35,000 times in total. If running speed is constant throughout a marathon, it's likely that heart rate will gradually rise as it has to gradually work harder to supply blood to the muscles for energy, and to the skin to maintain body temperature. To meet the demands of a marathon, between the start and the finish the heart will have pumped around 5000 litres (8800 pints) of blood around the body.

THE LUNGS

With a surface area of 50–75m² (540–800ft²) – or half of a tennis court – the lungs are called into immediate action as soon as a marathon starts. Large volumes of air rapidly and continuously enter and leave the lungs, 21 per cent of which consists of oxygen.

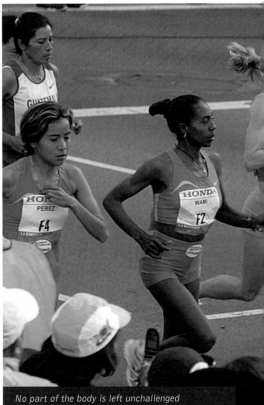

No part of the body is left unchallenged by the demands of running a marathon.

Some of this oxygen passes through the thin walls of the alveoli – microscopic sacs at the periphery of the lungs, where it enters the bloodstream and is pumped to the muscles by the heart.

THE LIVER

The liver is an energy store, which is used to top up and replenish the muscles stores of glycogen during the race. On the start line, most runners will have 100–120g (4–5oz) of glycogen in their livers, but by the finish this reserve will be virtually empty. This is because liver glycogen enters the bloodstream as glucose before being transported to the muscles, where it is converted to muscle glycogen.

THE KIDNEYS

Once running starts, the blood supply to our kidneys falls to around 25 per cent of the level at rest, ensuring that the supply of blood to

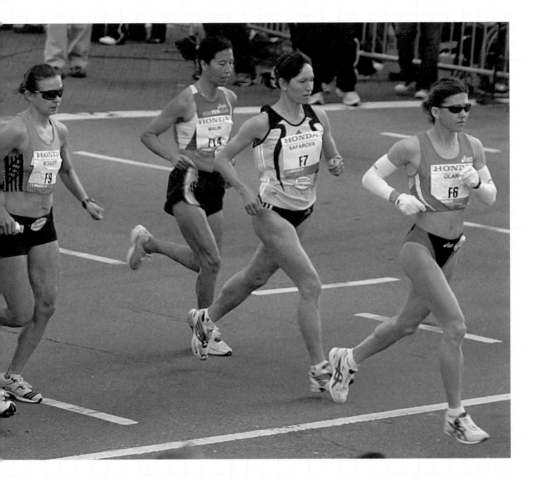

the muscles and brain can be maintained. Hormones are released that help to conserve fluid by restricting the kidneys' production of urine, although they still work hard during a marathon to filter and cleanse the blood of impurities and potentially harmful by-products of exercise.

THE STOMACH

Ideally there should be no solid food within the stomach when a marathon starts, since partially digested matter could cause stomach pains and discomfort. Once running commences, the supply of blood to the stomach reduces rapidly, so fluids or gels, rather than solid foods, are the most sensible way of refuelling and rehydrating during the race.

THE GUTS

Marathon running results in a shift of blood away from the guts, and partly as a result of

this, it is not uncommon for many runners to suffer from gut pains and disorders, often because food remains partially digested when the gun goes, or as a result of poor pre-race nutritional strategy. Fluid consumed during the race will still enter the gut and be absorbed by the bloodstream to help combat dehydration.

THE SKIN

Often overlooked as a vital organ, the skin is kept busy throughout the entire race. The rubbing and impact forces that are part and parcel of marathon running create friction that damages skin cells, leading to abrasions and blisters. At the same time, the skin is the critical site for the evaporation of sweat that keeps the body cool, preventing overheating and hyperthermia.

MARATHON PSYCHOLOGY

Marathons are physically tough, but can be mentally overwhelming. Understanding the psychology involved is essential if the finish line is to be reached successfully and enjoyably.

The physical challenge of marathon training and running is easy to quantify, and immediately apparent when runners are seen staggering and struggling over the last few miles. Yet ask any marathon runner, and they will tell you that the psychological challenge of a marathon can be as great, if not greater, than the physical one.

I have had experience of this myself, and it is all too easy to have a marathon run undone by the mental demons that produce doubt, anxiety and even panic as the prospect of the distance ahead becomes all consuming. However, the science of sports psychology provides a range of techniques to help runners prepare for, and complete, the distance. For example, during the race build-up, staying focussed on the race ahead is vital – it is all too easy to forget this at major marathons, where pre-race Expos and the excitement of the impending race day can become a big distraction. Sports psychologists recommend adopting a technique called 'visualisation', whereby you picture yourself running and finishing

'Nearly all runners will start a marathon with a personal goal – for some this is to finish, for others it is to run a good time.'

the race. When I have run the London Marathon with celebrities, I often suggest that they visualise themselves running past Buckingham Palace, turning into The Mall, and finishing the race in front of thousands of spectators. Visualising the finish of a marathon also works well as a motivational tool during training, and can act as a timely reminder of why the sacrifices of marathon preparation are being made.

Sports psychologists who have studied runners during a marathon have found

that elite runners use a technique called 'association', where they maintain a sharp awareness of their own body, and the physical factors that influence performance. They respond to changes in feelings of effort, and are acutely aware of the pace at which they are running. On the other hand, non-elite runners have been found to use a technique that at times can almost be a form of self-hypnosis known as 'dissociation'. This enables them to cut themselves off from feedback

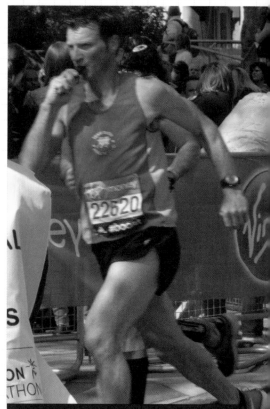

Marathons are never easy, and at some stage mental resilience will be needed to help overcome the miles and reach the finish.

and discomfort that they are experiencing – something that can be easier to do in mass marathons where cheering crowds and famous landmarks can act as a distraction from the effort of running.

In practice, I have found that most runners, regardless of ability, use a combination of both techniques, 'zoning in' to associate with their body, then 'zoning out' for a period of dissociation when things get tough, or when on-course distractions make this easier to do. This often happens subconsciously, with runners switching from one to the other as the race progresses.

Nearly all runners will start a marathon with a personal goal – for some this is to finish, for others it is to run a good time. Psychologists have found that one of the biggest mental challenges faced by marathon runners occurs when they start thinking that their goal is unobtainable – perhaps simply because they are having a bad run, or possibly thanks to injury. This can result in what I sometimes call the 'psychological crisis point' in a marathon – doubts creep in, and the challenge ahead can seem insurmountable. When the physical fatigue of the 18–20-mile point starts to become apparent, it is all too easy to become mentally overwhelmed by the 6–8 miles that are left, rather than focusing on the achievement of having already covered the bulk of the distance.

If things get tough – and they almost certainly will – resetting goals, aiming to complete and not compete, visualising the finish, and alternating from association to dissociation, are all successful ways of using the science – and art – of psychology to help reach the finish line.

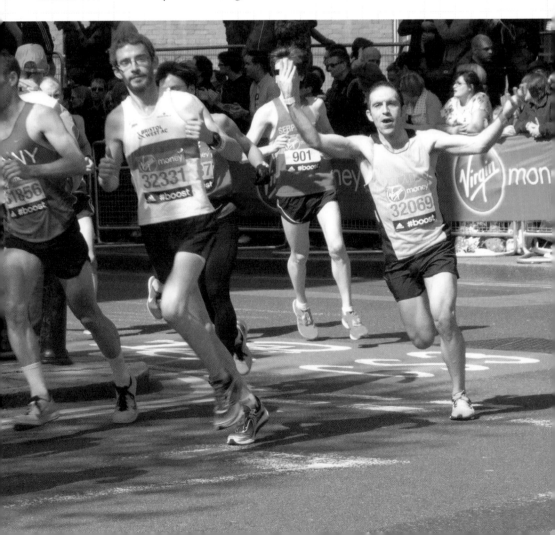

MARATHON NUTRITION

Marathon runners need energy. With poor refuelling, fatigue soon follows, but get it right, and your running will be supported by a plentiful supply of high-quality energy.

Consider a high-performance car – no matter how well tuned it is, if you put in the wrong fuel, it won't go well. Worse still, if you don't put in enough fuel, it will stop altogether. Training and running marathons is no different. Correct nutrition is vital if training, recovery and racing are to be optimised, giving a runner the best possible chance of completing the distance as quickly and as enjoyably as possible. We have already seen that most runners expend around 3000 calories when running a marathon, equivalent to a normal daily intake of energy for males. Most of this comes from carbohydrate stored in the muscle and liver as a substance called glycogen.

However, nutrition also needs to support training – someone typically running around 50 miles per week during their training will expend an additional 6000 calories on top of their normal weekly energy output – equivalent to an additional two days of food.

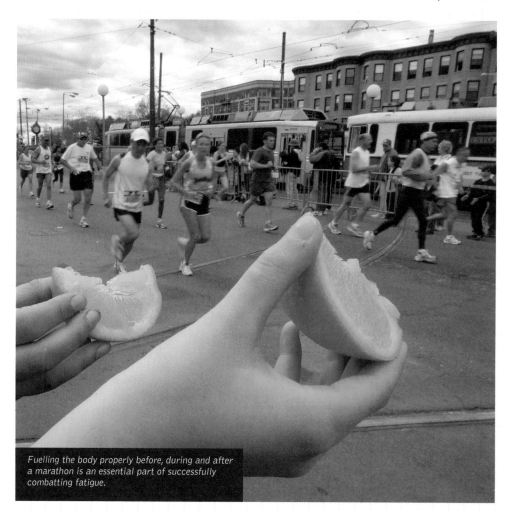

Fuelling the body properly before, during and after a marathon is an essential part of successfully combatting fatigue.

'...someone typically running around 50 miles per week during their training will expend an additional 6000 calories on top of their normal weekly energy output – equivalent to an additional two days of food.'

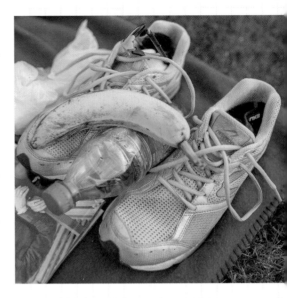

With all of us, if energy intake does not meet energy output, weight will be lost, initially from stores of fat, which can be a good thing since it reduces bodyweight and running thus requires less effort. However, constant weight loss for a long time can be damaging to health, and may lead to a loss of muscle – or protein – which reduces strength and increases the risk of injury and illness.

This extra demand for energy from marathon training needs to be matched by an increase in carbohydrate intake, particularly during the recovery period after a run. An enzyme called glycogen synthase converts carbohydrate to glycogen, and this is at its most active during the first few hours after strenuous exercise when glycogen has been depleted. Consequently, consuming carbohydrate as soon as possible after a run is important since this accelerates the recovery process by rapidly restoring the reduced energy stores.

The Ancient Greeks would have fed the original marathon runner Pheidippides a diet high in protein. Today, we know that this would probably have slowed him down since it would have taken a long time to digest, possibly have resulted in stomach cramps, and would have made only a limited contribution to the energy needed to run from Sparta to Athens. However, more recently, scientists have shown that combining some protein with the carbohydrates consumed after a long run can help to promote recovery, mainly by enhancing the muscles' uptake of glycogen. That said, runners who think that eating lots of protein will help them gain strength will be misleading themselves – many research studies have found that the best way to gain strength is through a combination of training and a modest protein intake.

There are some who see marathons, and the training that accompanies them, as a means of losing weight. This is not a good policy, since the only way to lose weight properly is by creating an energy deficit where intake is less than expenditure, and this is not good for runners, who need energy to train and race effectively. Carbohydrate should be the focal point of a marathon runner's diet, but it is important to be sensible and not overeat, based on the false assumption that running is an

'... runners who think that eating lots of protein will help them gain strength will be misleading themselves – many research studies have found that the best way to gain strength is through a combination of training and a modest protein intake.'

excuse to eat more and snack frequently. When you start training, you may actually gain some weight as muscle mass increases in the legs, but once you are settled into a training routine, your bodyweight should remain constant, with only limited fluctuations.

Crucial to staying healthy and fuelled for marathon training and racing is a varied, balanced diet, high in carbohydrate and fresh fruit and vegetables, which will ensure that you consume all the vitamins, minerals and energy that are needed to support your marathon-running lifestyle.

MARATHON HYDRATION

Knowing how to stay hydrated is crucial for marathon success. Get it wrong, and the consequences are serious and potentially dangerous.

Scientists have shown that the two biggest challenges faced by marathon runners of all abilities are the loss of fuel and fluid. While the loss of fuel only starts to impact on performance during the latter stages of the race, losing fluid can quickly lead to dehydration and have an early impact on performance. If dehydration persists and gets worse, body temperature will rise and the consequences are overheating, and a condition called hyperthermia, which could result in death.

Marathon runners need to sweat – the evaporation of sweat is the body's main defence against a rise in core temperature. But sweating results in the loss of body fluid,

'Hot and humid conditions will present more of a challenge to hydration status than cooler ones - the heat makes it harder for the body to stay cool, while humidity makes it more difficult for it to sweat efficiently.'

and experiments have found that once more than 2 per cent of bodyweight has been lost as a result of sweating, physical and mental performance suffer. Closer examination of runners during races has found that in hot and humid conditions, sweat rates can exceed 3 litres (5¼ pints) an hour, with rates of 1–2 litres (1¾–3½ pints) an hour not uncommon. Since the 2 per cent weight-loss threshold is just 1.5kg (3.3lb) for a 75kg (11st 8lb, or 165lb) runner, it is easy to see that dehydration is a much earlier threat in a marathon than the loss of energy. Even on cool days, runners still sweat, and we also lose moisture with every breath as we exhale, so maintaining the correct state of hydration before, during and after long training runs and a marathon is essential.

It is hard to believe, but in the early days of marathon racing, alcohol was seen as an ideal means of hydrating, and the 1904

Olympic Champion, Thomas Hicks, was given copious quantities of alcohol during his run. Today, our scientific knowledge of marathon hydration has advanced enormously, based on the development of rehydration drinks for individuals suffering from debilitating and dehydrating diseases such as cholera. In 1965, medics working with the University of Florida's American Football team – the Gators – developed a drink containing carbohydrate and electrolytes to aid the team's performance (electrolytes support the function of the muscles and nerves, and are lost when we sweat, so their replacement is crucial when sweat rates are high). This drink became the

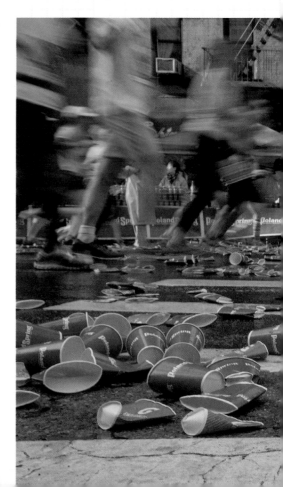

sports drink 'Gatorade' and sparked a series of research studies into the effect of similar drinks on endurance performance.

Not surprisingly, research studies found that these drinks were beneficial for marathon runners, improving endurance performance and cognitive function by replacing the fluids and electrolytes lost in sweat. Scientists discovered that with an optimum blend of carbohydrate – 4–8g of carbohydrate per 100ml (1/8–1/4oz of carbohydrate per 3.4fl oz) – and electrolytes in the form of sodium and potassium, running performance improved and fatigue was delayed. These drinks are quickly absorbed into the bloodstream, providing rapid replacement of energy, fluid and electrolytes. They became known as 'isotonic' drinks, and are now widely used, alongside water, in many marathons.

Even with fluid on course, most runners will finish a marathon dehydrated to a greater or lesser extent. Weight decrease of 4–5kg (8.8–11lb) at the end of a marathon is not uncommon, much of which will be due to a loss of fluid. Hot and humid conditions will present more of a challenge to hydration status than cooler ones – the heat makes it harder for the body to stay cool, while humidity makes it more difficult for it to sweat efficiently. Sweat that evaporates is most effective in losing heat, but in humid conditions sweat tends to drip rather than evaporate. The body reacts by producing more sweat, hence more fluid is lost and hydration becomes even more important.

Correct and efficient hydration is one of the most important components of marathon success, enabling the body to maintain its core temperature and preventing overheating. The science of hydration has made significant advances, and is now an integral part of the advice given to runners before marathons, and the on-course fluid offered to runners during a race.

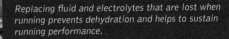

Replacing fluid and electrolytes that are lost when running prevents dehydration and helps to sustain running performance.

SLEEP

Why waste time sleeping when there is marathon training to be done? Well think carefully, because sleep is as crucial as a long run when it comes to marathon preparation.

Most of us spend approximately one-third of our lives asleep, and it is easy to view this as time that is 'wasted', with little benefit for marathon training or racing. However, sleep is an essential part of a runner's training, and is the time when many of the physiological adaptions to the stimulus of training takes place.

The human 'body clock' is regulated by a series of cycles known as the 'circadian rhythm', which determines areas such as digestion, hunger, body temperature and heart rate, as well as the time of day when we sleep. Sleep scientists have found that we have a series of sleep phases each lasting approximately 90 minutes, which initially take us into alternating periods of deeper and lighter sleep, before gradually emerging to a lighter pre-awakening stage characterised by rapid eye movement, or REM.

It is during the deeper, non-REM phases, where sleep does most to help to support marathon runners. One of the first things to occur is the redistribution of blood supply, with over 40 per cent of the blood that normally goes to the brain during waking hours diverted to the muscles. At the same time, hormones are released that help with the repair and growth of tissues, something that is essential after a long or intensive run or race. One of the main hormones that is released is human growth hormone, which plays an essential part in rebuilding and developing the proteins that constitute the muscle fibres that will have been repeatedly exposed to the rigours and stimulus of running. Muscle- and liver-glycogen stores will also be replenished, ensuring that energy reserves are at full capacity in time for the next run.

There is also evidence to suggest that sleep helps to support the body's immune system, something that is crucial if illness and infections are to be avoided. While asleep, the body releases proteins called cytokines. Some of these help to promote sleep, while others are important in the fight against inflammation and infection, and to combat the physical

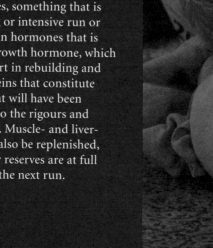

stresses that are caused as a result of marathon training.

Scientists and medical practitioners often recommend exercise during the daytime as a means of enhancing sleep quality, since the body responds to the need to recover and repair by increasing sleeping time and quality. However, since sleep involves a reduction in heart rate, core temperature and blood pressure, it is not advisable to finish a run just before going to bed, because the residual effects of an elevated metabolic rate will make it much harder to fall asleep.

While there are clear and unequivocal benefits from sleep for marathon runners, continuous sleep loss can be a major issue, with the risk of injury, illness and fatigue

all increasing. The amount of sleep that we require varies from one person to another, with 7–8 hours being the norm for most adults.

So sleep is as much a part of a marathon runner's preparation and training as a long run, and without the restorative effects of sleep it would be impossible to train effectively and complete 26.2 miles. Nevertheless, few runners get a sound night's sleep before a marathon, due to the combined effects of anxiety and the need to wake at an early hour to get to the start line. While it is easy to panic if you are not sleeping well on the night before a race, I have never yet seen a marathon runner fall asleep on the course, and if you do, there are plenty of other runners and spectators to wake you back up!

Sleep is part of the crucial recovery process, and a time when the body adapts to the stimulus of training.

THE PERFECT RUNNING STYLE

Moving forwards as quickly and as effortlessly as possible is a goal that all runners strive to achieve. But looks can be deceiving and the perfect style may not suit everyone.

Whereas physiologists get excited about marathon runners' ability to utilise oxygen, biomechanists are more concerned with the analysis and development of optimum running style. In achieving the basic objective of running in a forward direction, the body's limbs act in a manner that creates many sub-movements, which can frequently be opposed to the direction of travel. The scientific term for the movements created by the running body is 'momentum', which is a function of mass and speed. While the predominant momentum of the runner will be forwards, the alternate movements created by the left and right legs moving forwards for each stride cause some rotational momentum, which is countered by movements of the arms to stop the body twisting. This is why each stride with the right leg is accompanied by a forward swing of the left arm, and vice versa.

However, no two runners will achieve this basic running style in the same way. Differences in weight, height, running speed and limb length all affect style, and subconsciously most tend to adopt a style that suits them. It is worth reminding ourselves that the human body is designed to run – along with walking it is a natural form of movement for us. While some runners may feel that they need to modify their running technique, this rarely seems to produce significant benefits, and in some cases can even be counter-productive. One of the greatest marathon runners of all time, Paula Radcliffe, had a style that many analysts would say was

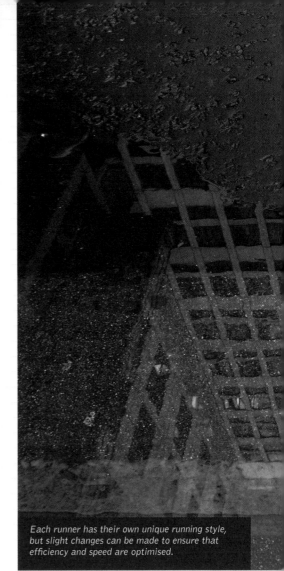
Each runner has their own unique running style, but slight changes can be made to ensure that efficiency and speed are optimised.

less than perfect, yet she was capable of running a marathon faster than any woman in history, and adopted a style that suited herself, not the scientists.

One area of running style that has generated a great deal of interest is the point of impact between the ground and the leg, often referred to as 'foot strike'. While the point of foot strike for sprinters is always the very front of the foot, since they drive forwards to produce maximum power and speed, endurance runners tend to favour foot strike at the rear, beneath their heel. However, some will strike further forwards towards the mid-foot, or in rarer cases the forefoot is the

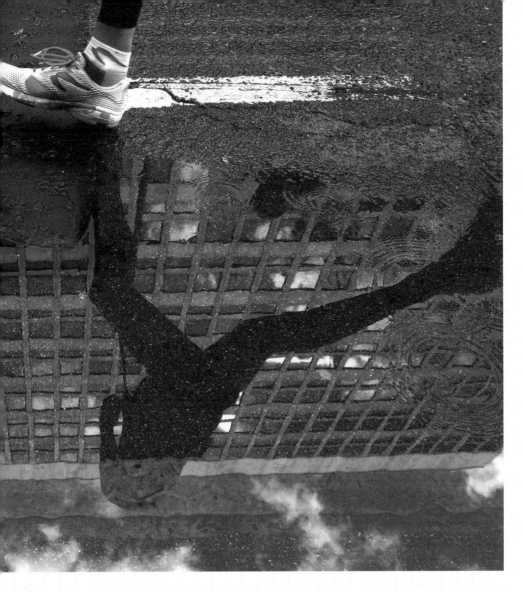

point of impact. Some scientists and coaches suggest that mid-foot and forefoot running is more natural, reflecting a style that precedes the development of today's highly cushioned running shoes. But there are also sports-injury specialists who suggest that mid-foot and forefoot running places stresses on the small bones of the mid-foot – the metatarsals – which could lead to fractures and injury.

The second area of foot strike that has received focus is the angle at which the foot hits the ground. Most runners tend to impact with the outer edge of their foot – the heel makes contact and they then tend to 'roll' in towards the mid-foot and

forefoot, before pushing off at the end of the stride. But some runners 'over-pronate' – this is when the foot rolls in too far, creating stresses on the muscles, tendons and ligaments that could lead to injury.

Our running styles are unique, and involve the management of energy in a way that moves the body forwards as quickly and as efficiently as possible. While it may be possible to change a runner's style, this should only be done in the sure knowledge that doing so will either reduce the risk of injury, or the amount of effort that is needed. If it doesn't look good, it doesn't have to be fixed!

THE SCIENCE OF RACE TACTICS AND STRATEGIES

You may have a target time, but have you got a strategy to achieve it? Planning your race from the start, and reacting to the conditions, is essential for success.

Most runners stand on the marathon start line with a target time in mind and with many months of dedication and hard training behind them. Yet all of the plans and effort can be undone with poor race tactics, so having a strategy to cope with the changing demands of the race is essential, and is something that every runner, whether elite or recreational, has to consider.

From a scientific perspective, running an even pace at a constant, tolerable speed makes most sense. As we have already discussed, selecting a pace that enables your body to burn a combination of fat and carbohydrate helps to spare the all-important muscle-glycogen stores so that your speed can be sustained until the finish. The problem with this strategy is that it leaves no room for error, and it's all too easy to see

> '**Setting off too quickly in an attempt to get time 'in the bank' should be avoided, since this burns glycogen rapidly, and risks a significant drop in pace towards the end.**'

a target time slipping away if pace drops by even a small amount towards the end of a race. Furthermore, in mass events where the roads are crowded, I have found that sustaining a constant speed during the latter stages can be difficult when others around you are slowing.

Some runners aim for a 'negative split' – the term given when the second half is faster than the first. While psychologically it can feel great to be running faster while those around you are slowing, this again causes problems in crowded races, and puts a lot of pressure on your ability to dig deep and run faster after you have already completed

a significant distance. It is a tactic best used by elite runners who have the experience, fitness and uncrowded roads to accelerate away from their rivals as the race unfolds.

Setting off too quickly in an attempt to get time 'in the bank' should be avoided, since this burns glycogen rapidly, and risks a significant drop in pace towards the end, wiping out the faster pace at the start.

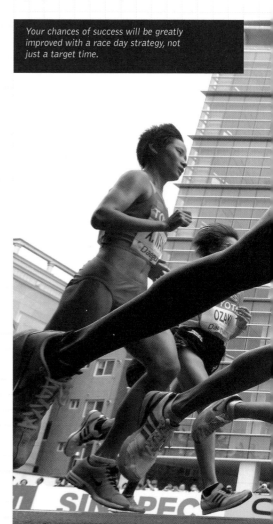

Your chances of success will be greatly improved with a race day strategy, not just a target time.

MYTH: **MARATHON RUNNING IS ALL IN THE MIND**

It's not unknown to hear coaches and runners state that the mental aspect of marathon running is tougher than the physical one, but in reality this only really applies to runners who are already well trained and experienced at completing the marathon distance. Of course the mental aspect of marathon running is crucial – both at the start to help overcome the seemingly immense distance that there is to cover, and at the end to overcome the pain and fatigue that build up – but physical conditioning will always remain at the heart of preparation for a marathon; if it were just down to mental resilience then there would be no need to invest in the long months of training and hard work.

The cardiovascular system needs to be capable of transporting large volumes of blood and oxygen to the muscles, while the legs need to be able to sustain many thousands of strides, and to withstand the impact forces that occur each time a foot hits the ground. Developing a level of fitness that helps the body burn fat rather than carbohydrate, thus sparing limited stores of muscle glycogen, is essential, and mental resilience alone is no substitute for a lack of training. Of course, that said, marathon training also requires mental toughness, and a determination to complete the necessary training sessions and lonely miles of running. Ideally, running a marathon relies on physiology and psychology, and together they provide the perfect combination to support completion of the distance.

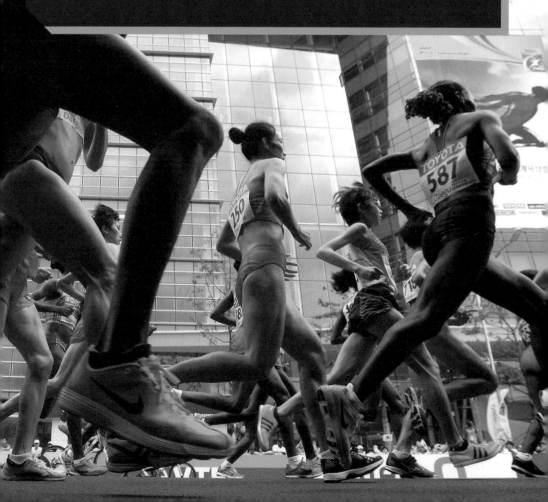

I find that a sensible strategy is to set an early speed that allows for a 5–8 per cent drop in pace in the second half of the race. So, for someone aiming for a 4-hour marathon, this means a first half in around 1 hour 56 minutes, so that the target can be reached with a 2 hour 4 minute second half.

Marathons are constantly changing, and one of the biggest factors to take into account when planning your strategy is the weather. I have stood on the start line shivering in the early morning cold, only to find myself sweltering under a baking sun some 3–4 hours later. Check the weather forecast before the race starts, and take into account the potential for altering conditions as the race unfolds. The wind is another factor to consider – running in a group can help to shield you from the force of the wind, although it is important to maintain a pace that is right for you, not others. Race topography should also be taken into account – if the course has hills towards the end, or is downhill at the start, plan your pace and tactics accordingly.

The trend for elite runners to have pacesetters is now commonplace for recreational runners, with many mass races having clearly identifiable pacers who set the speed for a range of target times. These work well and can take much of the psychological pressure off marathon running, but selecting the right pacer is critical if you are to avoid going too fast or too slow.

Successfully completing a marathon needs planning and thought. This requires a target time and – crucially – a strategy and tactical plan to achieve it.

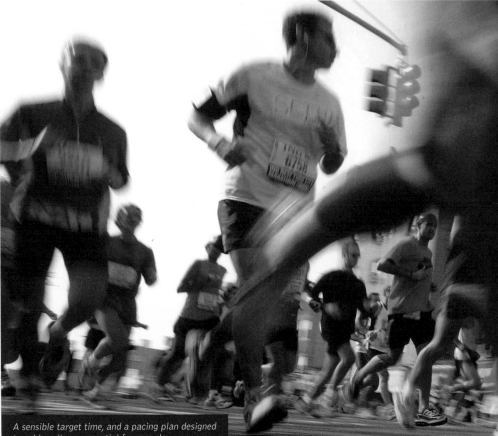

A sensible target time, and a pacing plan designed to achieve it, are essential for race day.

MYTH: *SMALLER RUNNERS ARE FASTER*

Most elite marathon runners are light in weight, and it is rare to see top marathon runners who have a large physique. Every extra kilogram of weight needs to be carried around the course, and that in turn needs more energy and oxygen. A runner weighing 55kg (8st 9lb, or 121lb) needs much less energy to complete 26.2 miles than one weighing 85kg (13st 5lb, or 187lb), and the physique of the best marathon runners in the world tends to favour individuals who are quite short, lightweight, with very little body fat, and a relatively long stride length.

However, that does not mean that individuals with a different stature and physique cannot complete the distance, and complete it quickly. Taller people tend to have a long stride length, and if two runners have the same stride rate, but one

has a stride length that is just 1cm (½in) longer than the other, the runner with the longer stride will finish around 350m (380 yards) ahead of the runner with the shorter stride. Taking fewer strides reduces stresses placed on the body, and enables the miles to be covered quickly and efficiently. However, carrying extra weight – particularly body fat – is a disadvantage when it comes to marathon running. It requires extra energy, the extra fat makes no contribution to performance or metabolism, and is likely to place more stress on the body's heat-control mechanisms.

Marathon runners come in all shapes and sizes, and all have the capacity to run 26.2 miles well, and quickly, provided that their physique is underpinned by crucial physiological adaptations as a result of many miles of training.

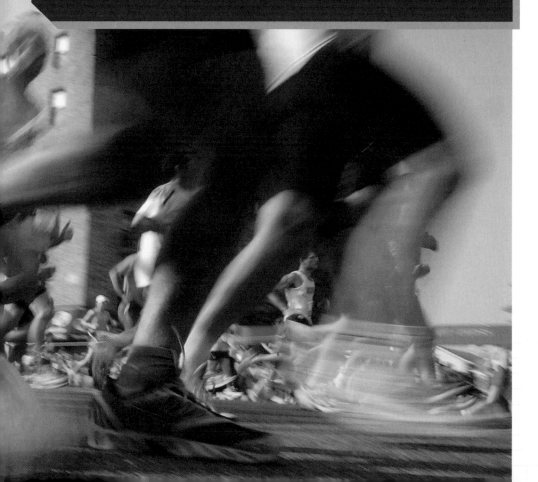

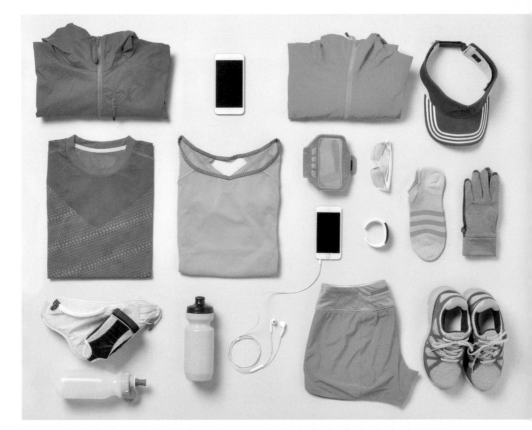

THE SCIENCE OF RUNNING KIT

Marathons are not fashion parades, but wearing the right clothing is as crucial for runners as it is for highly paid catwalk models. Science meets practicality when it comes to marathon style.

Over the years, manufacturers and scientists have invested considerable time and money into the development of clothing and footwear designed to make marathon running easier and faster. It is hard to quantify the extent to which these developments have helped, and how much better they are than the string vest, cotton shorts and leather shoes that were the common attire of marathon runners in the 1950s and 1960s. Performance enhancement and injury prevention are integral to the science of running kit, but alongside these there is the fundamental need for a runner to feel good, and comfortable, in whatever they choose to wear.

SHOES

This is the area where there has been the greatest investment and advances in recent years. The use of lightweight fabrics for the uppers, to replace the heavier leather of the past, has been complemented with cushioned soles that are designed to reduce and distribute the impact forces generated by each stride. Shoes have been adapted to meet the needs of different running styles, or to support runners who suffer from biomechanical issues such as

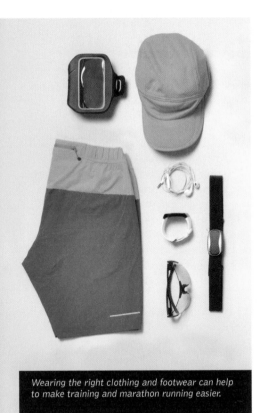

Wearing the right clothing and footwear can help to make training and marathon running easier.

pronation. Further individualisation comes with the use of orthotics – inserts that are placed within a shoe to minimise the risk of injury. Recently, there has been a move towards 'natural' running shoes, which keep the front and rear of the foot in a flatter position than shoes that elevate the heel with cushioning, based on the theory that this encourages a more natural forefoot running style.

SOCKS

Alongside the design of lightweight, seamless socks that combine comfort with a reduced risk of abrasions and blisters, the main focus of scientists has been the development of compression socks, which fit tightly around the foot and lower leg. The science of compression garments has two main strands – the first is that by compressing the muscles, it is possible to force blood to flow deep into the muscle, improving blood supply and the removal of lactic acid. I am not yet convinced that this is the case, since the additional

tightness may constrict rather than improve blood flow, which in turn is governed by heart rate and cardiac output. The second strand is injury prevention – calf-muscle strains are common among runners, and after personally experiencing these on a regular basis, I found that the use of compression socks helped enormously. To understand why, I focussed on the impact forces that occur with each stride, and the vibrations that these send through the leg muscles. Any slight tear or strain will be made worse with each vibration, but if these vibrations can be controlled through the stabilising effect of compression socks, it supports their use for injury prevention.

SHORTS AND TOP

Being light in weight and comfortable are the main assets these garments should possess, and when this is complemented with the scientific development of material that helps to quickly remove sweat from the skin, there should be gains in performance. However, it is worth remembering that for sweat to achieve its primary function – heat loss – evaporation, not removal, is crucial. Lightweight shorts and traditional running vests remain viable, highly functional options for most runners. The exposure of skin – and sweat – to the external environment greatly improves sweat evaporation and thermoregulation. Covering up with long sleeves, long shorts and compression garments will only serve to compromise the heat-loss process. For some runners, however, wearing long sleeve tops and running tights can offer a comfortable option and may reduce the risk of chafing. Providing clothing has been tried in training and feels good without adding weight and heat, it should be good to run in.

SPORTS BRAS

Support and comfort are critical for female marathon runners, and there has been a significant amount of research into the development of supportive bras that reflect the individual characteristics of women and breast sizes. Supportive and lightweight, a good sports bra is essential for all female marathon runners.

THE SCIENCE OF OLDER RUNNING

Marathons defy age. There are few other sports where older competitors can continue to enjoy success, refocus, and train, and in which ageing becomes an opportunity, not a threat.

Ageing is inevitable, and with it comes a gradual decline in running performance. But for many marathon runners, the process brings new opportunities, and the chance to set new goals and times that may be surprisingly similar to those set many years in the past.

One of the key physiological determinants of marathon success is a runner's maximum oxygen uptake, or VO2 max. Scientists have found that for most, this peaks in the early to mid-20s, then gradually declines with age. For those who lead a sedentary lifestyle with little or no exercise, this decline can be as high as 10–12 per cent per decade, but for runners who train regularly, the decline can be as low as 5 per cent a decade. But for someone starting out as a marathon runner late in life, it is possible to improve maximum oxygen uptake to a level higher than that ever achieved in younger days, since it will only peak in the 20s if combined with regular training at that time. I have worked with some marathon runners who are fitter and healthier in their 50s and even 60s than they have been at any time previously, simply by adopting a lifestyle of training and healthy nutrition.

'Ageing should not be seen as a reason to despair, but instead as a challenge that can be met with sensible training, and embraced by setting new goals and target times.'

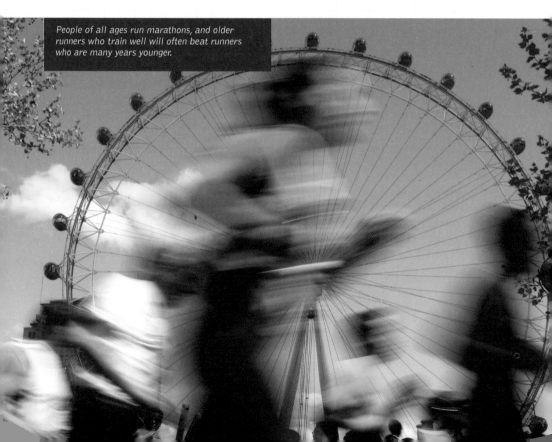

People of all ages run marathons, and older runners who train well will often beat runners who are many years younger.

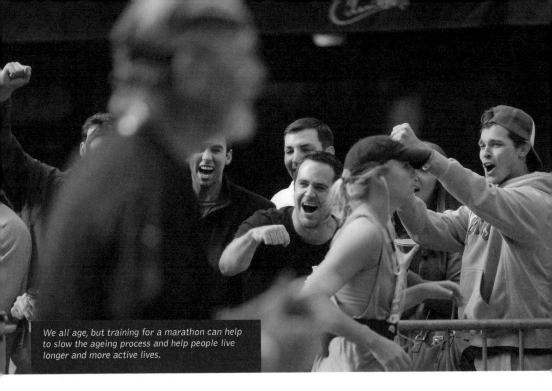

We all age, but training for a marathon can help to slow the ageing process and help people live longer and more active lives.

While training and running marathons will not halt the ageing process, there is plenty of scientific evidence to suggest that it will slow down the process, allowing for a long and productive running career.

Along with the decline in oxygen uptake, we also lose muscle mass and strength as we age. Scientists call this muscle loss 'sarcopenia', which can be up to 1 per cent of total muscle mass a year. However, as with oxygen uptake, the reduction can be slowed with training, consequently sustaining the strength and power that are needed to produce faster times.

Ageing should not be seen as a reason to despair, but instead as a challenge that can be met with sensible training, and embraced by setting new goals and target times. A look at the world-best age-category times for marathons gives an exciting insight into the capability of older runners. 50-year-old men have run marathons in close to 2 hours 20 minutes, with women of the same age close to 2 hours 30 minutes. Even at 70 years of age, we see times of sub-3 hours for males, and close to 3 hours 30 minutes for females, while at 80, the male best time is around 3 hours 15 minutes, and the female best time is

4 hours 10 minutes. All of these are times that many far younger runners would aspire to and be delighted to achieve.

Closer examination of these age-best times indicates that those who achieve them as veteran runners were almost certainly good, but not elite, runners in their earlier careers. This suggests that there are many current recreational and club runners who have the capacity to achieve great performances and times as they age, provided that they remain healthy and in regular training. While it is inevitable that the media will focus on world-record times that get ever closer to breaking the 2-hour barrier for a marathon, I think there is huge excitement and potential in the times that could be set by older runners in the future. We know from their times and laboratory data what today's elite runners are currently capable of. So far few, if any, have sustained their training and lifestyle into later years. But if they did, and based on the body's capacity to slow the ageing process as a result of training, the scientific data suggests that one day in the future, we could see an 80-year-old man running a marathon in under 2 hours 40 minutes, with an 80-year-old female not far behind in under 3 hours!

Marathon runners come from all backgrounds and could be novices or experienced runners, who gain satisfaction and fitness by training for and completing the distance.

MYTH: *MARATHON RUNNERS AGE QUICKER*

Marathon running has had a bad reputation for longevity since Pheidippides dropped dead after running 26 miles from Sparta to Athens in 490BC. This reputation is not helped by the commonly held image of many elite runners, who often appear underweight and anything other than healthy. Sadly, but inevitably, when there are fatalities during mass-marathon events, the media focuses on the negative impact and dangers of marathon running. This has led to some within the media and medical communities suggesting that marathons are harmful, put runners at high risk, and create intolerable stresses and strains on vital organs, bones, muscles tendons and ligaments that can at its worst put the runner at risk, and at best result in premature ageing.

Of course if you do too much of anything, and fail to prepare sensibly, you could do yourself harm. However, the vast majority of scientific evidence shows that the training and lifestyle adopted by marathon runners has huge positive health benefits, greatly reducing the potential risk of many life-threatening, and indeed life-ending, illnesses. Blood pressure and cholesterol are lowered, the calories burned reduce body fat and the risk of obesity, and the chances of heart attack, stroke and diabetes are lessened. While it is hard to state categorically that marathon runners live longer than non-marathon runners, it is likely that an activity that can be continued well into the latter stages of life will greatly improve the quality of that life, and act as a great way of preventing illnesses and catastrophic events.

MYTH: *YOU NEED A PERFECT RUNNING STYLE*

We all like to look good whatever we do, and running is no exception. But running styles are like fingerprints: no two runners are the same, and while running may appear to be simple – just putting one foot in front of the other quickly – it also involves a complex interaction of forces, limb movements, and momentum. All of these must operate together and as efficiently as possible so that running is as effortless as possible, while putting minimal stress on the muscles, tendons, bones and joints.

It is not uncommon for a runner to appear to be ungainly, with movement patterns that are less than aesthetic to most observers. In these situations, the temptation to change a runner's style is great, but more often than not this style

suits them, and forcing changes that improve appearance can end up having a negative effect on performance. Of course if there are obvious issues, or repeated injury problems that can clearly be traced to a poor running style, then coaching and change will be of benefit. However, in most other cases, changing running style can often do more harm than good, and not necessarily yield the desired improvements in running performance.

Marathon running is not about appearances, it is about covering 26.2 miles by conserving energy and reducing fatigue. As runners tire, running style will change, and sustaining a consistent style throughout the distance is as important – if not more important – than the style itself.

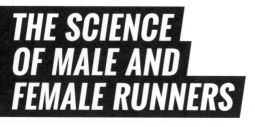

THE SCIENCE OF MALE AND FEMALE RUNNERS

Science and genetics play a part in determining whether marathon-running males or females come out on top. But that doesn't mean that the best can't beat the rest.

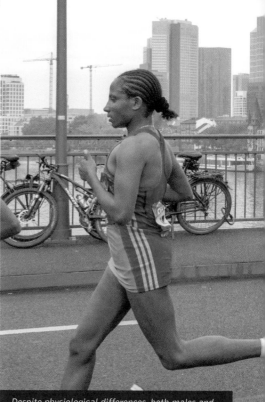

Despite physiological differences, both males and females are capable of running marathons, and many females will frequently beat male rivals.

When Paula Radcliffe broke the women's world record with a time of 2 hours 15 minutes in the 2003 London Marathon, she was not only the first female past the finish line, but in doing so also beat the vast majority of males in the same race. While this shows that great female runners are capable of running faster marathons than many males, the physiological reality is that our genetic characteristics give most males a natural marathon-running advantage over females.

The male physique tends to be bigger than that of females, with longer and larger bones, and greater muscle mass. This also results in larger lung volumes, presenting more opportunity for oxygen to enter the bloodstream. This is further aided by the fact that males have higher levels of haemoglobin than females. Haemoglobin is the constituent of the blood that carries oxygen from the lungs to the muscles, and having more means that there is greater capacity to get oxygen to the muscles to provide energy. On average, females have around 110g (41/2oz) of haemoglobin per 1 litre (1¾ pints) of blood, compared with 150g (6oz) per 1 litre (1¾ pints) for males.

The heart plays a crucial role in pumping oxygen-rich blood to the muscles, but the female heart tends to be slightly smaller than that of males. This means less blood and oxygen are pumped with each beat, or that the female heart needs to work harder (beat faster) to pump the same volume of

blood as a male heart. The combination of lower lung volumes, haemoglobin and heart size all contribute to females, on average, having a lower maximum oxygen uptake value than males. Since this is a key indicator of marathon-running success, it inevitably means that the majority of females will be starting a marathon at a physiological disadvantage when compared with males.

Lower levels of hormones such as testosterone also result in females tending to have a lower muscle mass than males, making it harder to produce the speed and power that are needed for faster running. Since marathons rely more on endurance than speed, this is not critical and is one reason why females can compete more effectively against males in endurance events as opposed to more explosive, power-based distances such as sprinting.

Paula Radcliffe and many other elite female marathon runners have shown that females can produce outstanding times,

MYTH: FEMALES COPE BETTER THAN MALES IN MARATHONS

Before 1984, women were not able to run marathons at the Olympics because the event was deemed 'too tough'. Fortunately, sense and science prevailed, to the extent that some scientists now suggest that females may be better suited to marathons than males, and that the female rather than the male world record may become the faster time. There are two reasons behind this myth. The first is down to energy reserves; genetically, women tend to have more body fat than men, and since fat means energy – and marathons need energy – it's easy to assume that women start with an advantage. This notion, however, is easy to dispel: carbohydrate is the main source of energy for marathons – and males tend to have greater carbohydrate stores than females. Even the lightest and leanest of men, with a body fat percentage of

around 7 per cent, will have 4kg (9lb) of body fat, equivalent to 36,000 calories – and most runners need fewer than 3000 calories to run 26.2 miles!

The second idea behind the myth is the rapid improvement in female marathon world-record times, suggesting that one day they will overtake their male counterparts. Closer analysis of the data, though, shows that this improvement is largely down to the late adoption of marathons by females, and that as rates of improvement slow, the gender gap in world-record times, in favour of males, will remain.

So, there are no physiological reasons to suggest that females are better able to cope with marathons than males. However, both sexes can equally manage the distance by preparing properly and racing at a sensible pace.

which are better than those of many males. Further down the field, there will always be a large number of good females, who combine their physiological capacity with training to excel and beat many good male runners. Females will continually beat males over marathons and shorter distances on a regular basis, but when averaged out across an entire race field, physiology and genetics will dictate that more males finish ahead of females than vice versa.

There are some areas where females may have an advantage over males. For example, their lighter bodyweight should place less stress on the lower limbs, and reduce the risk of injury. Some scientists have also suggested that females may be better able to maintain

'**There are some areas where females may have an advantage over males. For example, their lighter bodyweight should place less stress on the lower limbs, and reduce the risk of injury.**'

body temperature when running in the heat due to a greater surface-area-to-body-mass ratio, offering a larger surface from which heat can be lost.

Marathon running is one of the few sports in which males and females can compete in the same race, and there is no doubt that many female runners will continually beat males. But science and genetics have determined that males do have a physiological capacity that gives them a natural advantage over females.

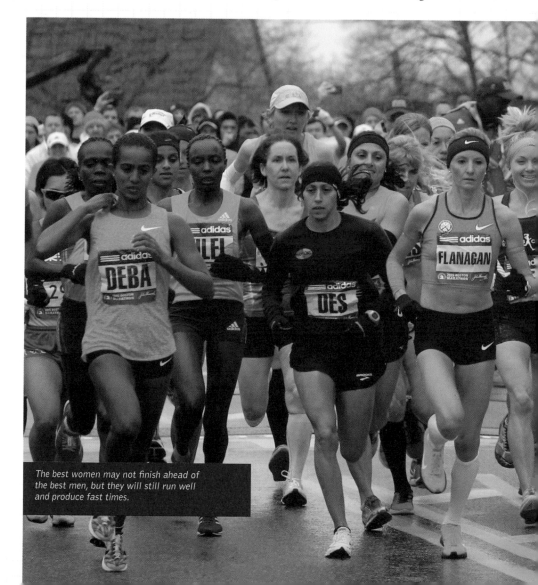

The best women may not finish ahead of the best men, but they will still run well and produce fast times.

MYTH: *IT TAKES SIX MONTHS TO TRAIN FOR A MARATHON*

The length of time needed to prepare for a marathon is very dependent on a runner's experience and starting point. For more experienced runners, conditioned to high weekly mileages and racing long distances, the preparation time can be quite short – often just a matter of a few weeks during which time the length of the weekly long run and weekly mileage are increased. For those after a fast time, this preparation time should be increased to encompass at least two to three months of heavy-endurance and speed-endurance training, long steady runs, and preparatory races, giving time for cardiovascular fitness and leg strength to adapt to the challenge of racing a marathon.

For novices, the preparation time is of course much longer. For someone starting from scratch and simply aiming to complete the distance, four to five months should be sufficient. There is a danger that if training time is longer, the willpower and motivation to train regularly will be eroded, and as the marathon nears, both the quantity and quality of training will decrease. I once worked with an individual who, with 100 days to go before the London Marathon, was 30kg (4st 10lb, or 66lb) overweight, smoked 30 cigarettes and day, and had high blood pressure and cholesterol. Under careful supervision, he embarked on a 100-day training programme, and successfully completed the marathon in a time just outside 5 hours. It transformed his life, and showed that marathons are possible provided that there is a sensible approach to training, realistic goals, and a determination to succeed.

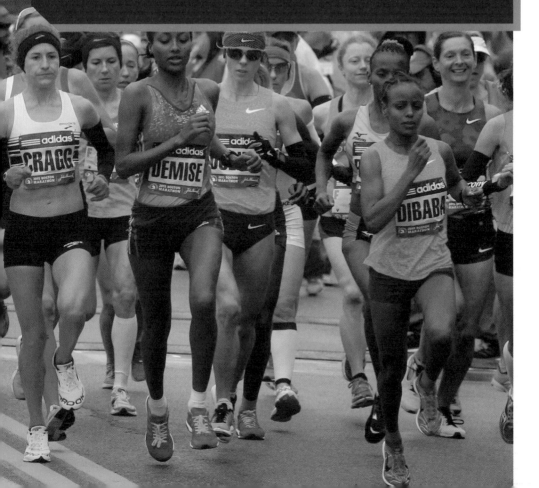

STRIVING TO IMPROVE

Completing your first marathon is a fantastic achievement. Running more, and improving your performance, is the next stage in the transition from being a marathon runner to becoming a marathon competitor.

Running your first marathon should be all about completing the distance. However, for runners aiming to revisit their marathon experience and compete in future events, competitive instinct and personal pride inevitably result in the desire to run faster. This means improving both the quantity and quality of your training, and supporting this with the changes in lifestyle and nutrition that underpin enhanced performance.

There are a number of scientific principles, outlined below, that apply to training for a marathon, and that need to be followed if improved performance is going to occur.

REGRESSION

Unfortunately, fitness quickly regresses if training time is missed. Studies have shown that after just three or four days of inactivity, fitness levels start to decline, so taking too much time off can quickly undo many of the gains that have come from hard-earned training miles.

SPECIFICITY

It may seem obvious, but marathons involve running. I once worked with someone who thought he could do all his marathon training on roller blades, since he was worried about the risk of knee injuries from running. Suffice it to say, he struggled after just 8 miles, and had to walk most of the remaining 18 miles to the finish. Running must constitute the bulk of marathon training, since it is the only way that the specific demands that marathons place on the body will be recreated.

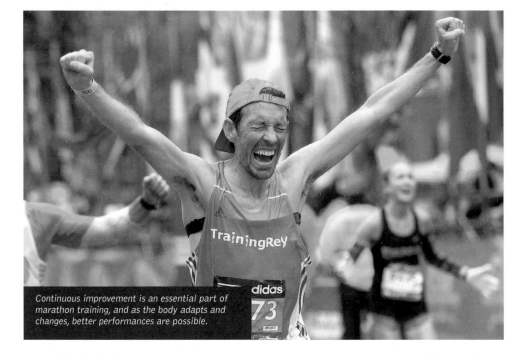

Continuous improvement is an essential part of marathon training, and as the body adapts and changes, better performances are possible.

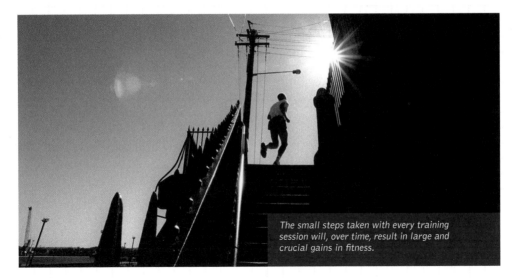
The small steps taken with every training session will, over time, result in large and crucial gains in fitness.

INTENSITY

Scientists have shown that marathon training needs to be at the right intensity if physiological adaptations are going to occur. If the intensity is too low, there will be few gains from the miles that have been covered. But if intensity is too high, fatigue, tiredness and even injury or illness could quickly arise. Laboratory studies have found that running at a pace that is just below the point where lactic-acid levels increase rapidly can bring significant benefits – for the majority of runners who are never able to have a lab test, this intensity is best described as 'tolerable discomfort', where a conversation can just be held.

PROGRESSION

Continually doing the same training run at the same speed will sustain fitness, but not improve it. Gradually increasing the duration, frequency and intensity of training will result in continual improvements in performance, but this needs to be achieved sensibly and steadily to avoid injury. Repetition running, often known as interval training, whereby runs include high-intensity bursts that are separated by periods of recovery, has been found to be a great way of increasing intensity and stimulating improvements in performance, without doing excessive mileage or extra training sessions.

RECOVERY

This is one of the most overlooked aspects of any training, but is essential if your body is going to adapt to the stimulus of training, and if continuous improvement is to occur. At least one rest day per week is vital for most marathon runners, and without this recovery time, fatigue, injury and illness will quickly follow.

MARGINAL GAINS

Underpinning training, improvements will only occur if other areas such as sleep, nutrition and hydration are not neglected. These become even more important as race day approaches, as does the psychological approach to race day, tactics and pacing. Individually, each of these may make only a small difference, but together, they can combine to have a significant difference on overall performance time. We all want to be the best that we can be in everything that we do, and marathon running is no exception. Progressing from 'marathon completer' to become a 'marathon competer' is a transition that not every runner can, or indeed wants, to make. But doing so opens up new challenges, and a different approach, that can yield great benefits and satisfaction from both training and racing.

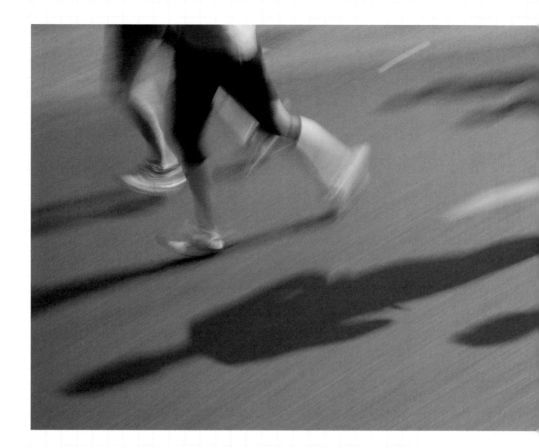

THE SCIENCE OF SPEED WORK

On the face of it, marathons are all about endurance. After all, 26.2 miles is a long way, and just keeping going at a constant pace is the main challenge faced by most runners. But that doesn't mean to say that speed work, and faster running, should not have an important role to play in marathon training.

The type of speed that marathon runners should focus on is speed endurance, rather than the raw pace of sprinters such as Usain Bolt. Our muscles consist of two main types of fibres: fast twitch and slow twitch, and it is the slow-twitch fibres that produce most of the energy for marathon running. These fibres contract at a relatively slow speed, but are slow to fatigue, so ideally suited for the sustained demands of marathons. In contrast, fast-twitch fibres contract rapidly, but also fatigue quickly so are more suited for sprinting.

Muscle-fibre type is largely determined at birth, and muscle biopsies have found that while sprinters have a predominance of fast-twitch fibres, marathon runners have a high proportion of slow-twitch ones. However, most runners also have a number of 'intermediate' fibres that share the characteristics of both slow- and fast-twitch muscle, and it is these fibres that runners are most likely to activate and develop when doing speed-endurance training.

Unlike steady endurance running, which occurs at speeds that do not cause

Although marathons are all about endurance, developing leg speed and strength helps the body to adapt and cope with the demands of running 26.2 miles.

MYTH: *YOU MUST TRAIN FOR FIVE OR SIX DAYS EACH WEEK*

There is no doubt that running a marathon requires a lot of training, and developing the strength and endurance that are needed to cope with the 26.2-mile distance is essential. Most elite runners have the luxury of lifestyles that enable them to train on a full-time basis, and this often includes more than one training session a day. Yet for most non-elite runners, training for a marathon has to be combined with work and family commitments, and the reality is that this makes it almost impossible to run on the five or six days per week that many marathon-training programmes advocate.

In an ideal world it would be great if this were not the case, but for many of us it holds true. Fortunately, it is certainly not impossible to complete a marathon on just two or three training sessions per week, provided that the quality of each session is high, and that one of them includes a long run that gradually increases in length to around 20–22 miles. A runner at the start of a marathon who has completed just two or three sessions per week, but with eight weeks where the weekly long run has extended from 15 to 22 miles, is likely to be far better prepared than a runner who has trained five times per week but whose longest run is only 18 miles. Recovery time is also crucial, and taking time off between runs allows the body to repair and adapt before the next training session.

a significant increase in lactic acid, speed-endurance training is at a higher intensity, generating faster leg speeds and lactic-acid production. This will normally consist of runs at a higher tempo, or interval training where shorter, faster bursts of running are interspersed with periods of recovery. Scientists have found that this is a great way of developing both leg speed and increasing maximum oxygen-uptake capacity. A good example of how speed-endurance training can be used to increase the intensity of a run is to switch a steady 5-mile run with five 1-mile runs, each at a higher speed than normal, with the 1 mile bursts separated by 2 minutes of slow jogging to recovery. Shorter, faster runs for around 20 minutes are beneficial, while many coaches and scientists also recommend doing races over distances from 10km to a half-marathon for which running speed is faster than marathon pace, since these are an alternative means of developing speed endurance.

As explained earlier, one of key ingredients for marathon success is being capable of running the race at a low relative exercise intensity, or percentage of maximum capacity. Many studies have found that speed-endurance work, when the body adapts to the production, tolerance and clearance of lactic acid, is an effective way of improving maximum capacity, or VO2 max. This means that running at a constant steady speed feels, and is, much easier since the pace produces less physiological stress once maximum capacity has been improved. So, while it is easy to assume that faster, shorter runs have little or no role to play in marathon training, nothing could be further from the truth, and their benefit is significant.

Speed-endurance running is the type of training that can quickly take a runner out of his or her comfort zone, and the results are impressive and the potential for improvement is significant. As with any type of training, it must only form one part of an overall training plan, but for many runners it can soon become the magic ingredient that transforms both training and performances.

MYTH: *YOU NEED TO RUN 40–50 MILES PER WEEK*

Marathon running has long been associated with runners who regularly run high weekly training mileages, and it is not uncommon to hear of marathon runners who complete over 100 miles per week when in heavy training. For many contemplating running a marathon, this knowledge can be daunting and off-putting. While a high weekly mileage is ideal for some, especially experienced runners with many years of running behind them, it will inevitably increase the risk of injury due to the repetitive forces and strains placed on the body. There is a fine line between completing the quantity and quality of training that is ideally needed for a marathon, and staying injury-free, something that is particularly true for novice runners who will not have developed the strength and resilience of those with more running-miles and experience.

As race day approaches, the length of the longest training run should increase, and thus the total weekly mileage will also extend. As a result, 30 miles per week is the minimum weekly distance that most runners will achieve, but for many this will occur towards the end of their marathon training, and not from the start. Attempting too many miles too quickly is one of the most common causes of fatigue and injury during marathon training, and it is far better to reduce weekly mileage while focussing on extending the length of the long weekly run, than it is to increase the weekly mileage too quickly and become injured.

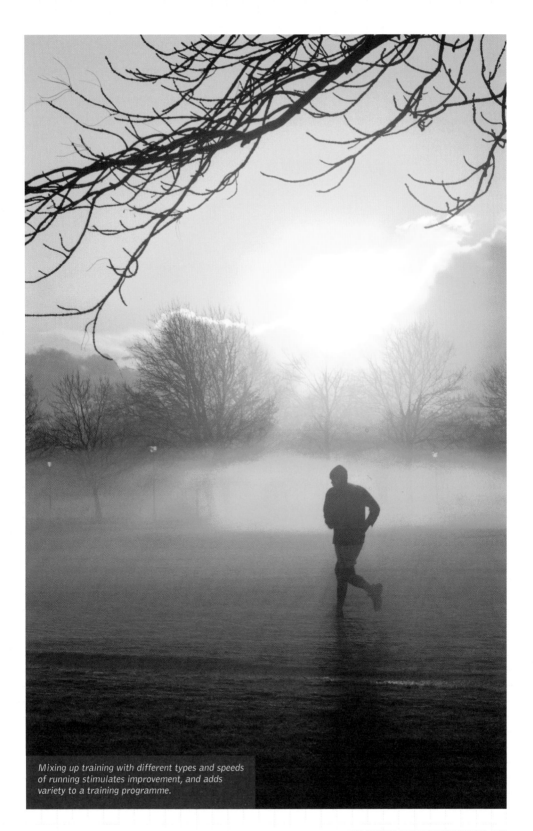

Mixing up training with different types and speeds of running stimulates improvement, and adds variety to a training programme.

SURVIVAL SCIENCE

When things go wrong, science can help. Using a range of science-based techniques, it is possible to survive the tough times, and successfully make it to the finish.

Inevitably in an event as long and as tough as a marathon, things don't always go quite according to plan. Although we have discussed areas where science can help to improve marathon performance, there are also many ways in which science can be utilised to help runners get through the tough times, survive the race, and make it to the finish line.

The most important thing to remember is that when things get tough, slowing down is not a disaster. It may mean that a target time will no longer be achieved, but it will reduce the physiological stress that the body is experiencing. When I have run marathons with celebrities, the tough times normally start from around 16 miles, and I have always supported them with a

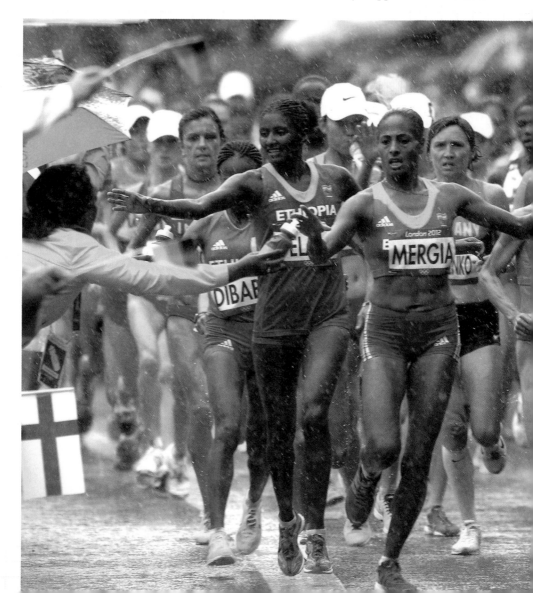

slight decrease in pace. However, wherever possible, we have still kept running. Pace reduction lowers heart rate and oxygen uptake, and allows the body to metabolise more fat, which is particularly helpful if glycogen stores are becoming low. After a short period of time, core temperature will also start to drop, which will be particularly welcome if the day is hot or humid. Pace reduction places the body into 'recovery mode', slowing things down and reducing the stress on the cardiovascular and thermoregulatory systems.

After a reasonable time, it may be possible to increase running speed again, but this is not essential, since the golden rule

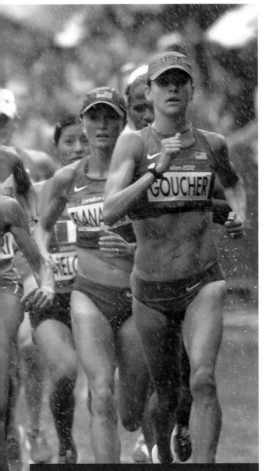

Sometimes things don't go to plan, but runners can use a range of scientific techniques to help them cross the finishing line.

when it comes to surviving and finishing is simply to keep going, and get through each mile. Wherever possible, try to avoid walking, since the change in gait from running to a walk can quickly lead to stiffness in the leg muscles, making it very hard to resume running again. Even when things get really hard, I advocate a shuffle rather than a walk, as I feel that both psychologically and physiologically this is better, even if the difference in speed is not that great.

Slowing down will also mean a shortening of stride length and a change in running style. There is scientific evidence to suggest that this could be beneficial, since it may allow the body to 'unlock' any remaining glycogen that remains in the muscles and muscle fibres that are brought into action by the gait change.

Sports psychology also has a critical role to play when things get tricky. I encourage runners to focus on what they have achieved, rather than what is still to come, and to visualise the feeling of euphoria when the finish line is crossed, and contrast that with the despondency that they will feel if they give up. In mass races, using the crowd for motivation and encouragement over the last few miles is also a useful survival tactic.

There is also a role for sports nutrition when it comes to surviving a marathon. The use of fluids and energy before and during a race is crucial, but when there are just a few miles to go, scientists have found that even the taste of something sweet can provide a boost to performance. It seems likely that sensors in the mouth detect the sweetness, and expect that this will soon lead to an energy boost. This gives an immediate lift, both psychologically and, it seems physically, even before any energy has reached the muscles.

So, even when things go wrong, science can come to the aid of weary marathon runners. There is a range of simple, science-based techniques that can be used to help runners get through those final challenging miles, and most importantly, ensure that the finishing line is crossed successfully.

BREATHING

Breathing is the essential first link in the provision of energy for marathons, and understanding, rather than changing, one of our most natural body functions is crucial.

While the legs do all the hard work during a marathon, it is the lungs that are essential if the legs are going to get the energy they need. We all need to breathe, but for marathon runners, the extraction of oxygen from air that enters the lungs, and the transport of this oxygen to the muscles, has to continue for the duration of a marathon at a rate that is often at least 10 times higher than at rest.

Breathing is the first stage of what is known as the respiratory system – the transport of air into and out of the lungs, depositing oxygen into the bloodstream, and removing one of the potentially harmful by-products of exercise, carbon dioxide. At rest, we take around 12 breaths per minute, and a total of around 6 litres (10½ pints) of air into and out of the lungs. Approximately one-fifth of this air is oxygen, and some – but not all –

is transported across the thin membranes of the lungs where it attaches to haemoglobin in the blood, and is pumped to the muscles by the heart.

However, when running starts, the muscles' demand for oxygen quickly rises, and breathing frequency consequently increases. So too does the volume of air taken into the lungs with each breath, which respiratory scientists call 'tidal volume'. At rest, tidal volume is around 500ml (17fl oz) per breath, rising to around 3 litres (5¼ pints) per breath during intensive exercise, although during marathons it is likely to be somewhat lower, at around 2 litres (3½ pints). Breathing frequency will rise to around 40 breaths per minute, so as a result the volume of air (known as the 'ventilation rate') going into and out of a marathon runner's lungs each

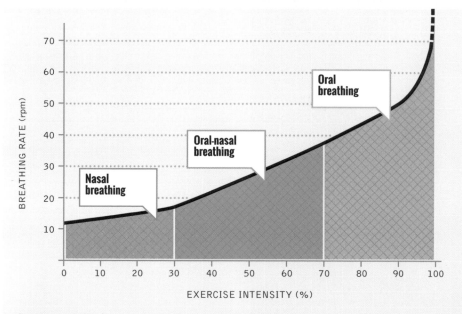

Breathing switches from nose to mouth as exercise intensity increases.

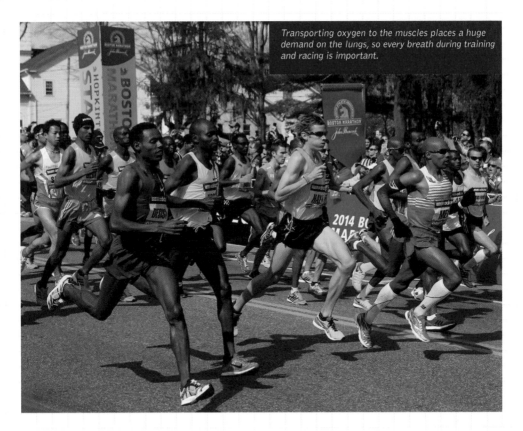

Transporting oxygen to the muscles places a huge demand on the lungs, so every breath during training and racing is important.

minute can easily reach 70–80 litres (123–140 pints). Over the duration of a 4-hour marathon, this could equate to 18,000 litres (31,675 pints) of air, and 10,000 breaths!

The dehydrating effect of breathing is often overlooked, but is significant and easy to demonstrate. Breathe out on to a cold pane of glass and the clouding that you see is moisture within the air condensing on the glass. With each breath, moisture will be lost, and while this is only secondary compared with the fluid lost from sweating, it can still play a part in dehydrating the body and drying the mouth and respiratory passages, even on the coldest of days.

Breathing takes place voluntarily, and fortunately it is not something we need to remind ourselves to do. The muscles responsible for raising the ribcage to draw air into the lungs are called the intercostal muscles, and just like any muscle in the body, they can tire. Training helps to develop these muscles in the same way that it develops the muscles of the legs, but as they inevitably fatigue, breathing

can become heavy and laboured, particularly towards the end of a race.

You will often see some runners lining up on the start line wearing nasal strips – simple devices that have become popular in recent years because they dilate the nostrils. Users claim that this nasal dilation makes breathing through the nose easier, which it probably does. However, scientists have shown that once exercise starts, and ventilation rates exceed 40 litres (70 pints) per minute, the body naturally resorts to the breathing method of least resistance, which is through the mouth. For the majority of sports, including marathon running, oral breathing is preferred to nasal breathing.

Breathing is something that we do naturally, and without thinking, and our bodies automatically adopt the intensity and type of breathing to suit the exercise we are doing. Attempting to change breathing patterns, or the way that we breathe, is not advisable, and more likely to result in poorer, rather than enhanced, performance.

RUNNING TECHNOLOGY

Running is simple, but running marathons is tough. Technological advances, when used properly, can help make the 26.2-mile journey a little bit easier.

There was a time when marathon runners simply put on a vest, shorts and a pair of leather shoes, trained outdoors on their own for mile after mile, then ran their race. While there is no doubt some people hanker for former times, advances in science and technology, combined with the growth of mass-participation marathon running, have changed the face of training and racing.

HEART RATE MONITORS

Alongside advances in kit and footwear, which have already been discussed (*see* pages 48–49), our greater understanding of the demands of marathon running, and the optimisation of training, has enabled science and industry to combine to help make training easier and more effective. One of the most common aids used by runners is the heart rate monitor, and we will discuss their application further in Section Two (*see* page 98). They help runners to judge the intensity of their training, and some even use them when racing. There is a danger that their usage can border on excessive, with runners paying more attention to their heart rate than to how their body feels. I normally suggest that runners use them as a guide, not a bible, and simply allow them to provide reassurance that their training is on track. Their use is complicated by the fact that even when running speed is constant, heart rate can gradually creep

upwards, particularly when conditions are hot since the heart has to work harder to pump blood to the skin to keep cool.

INDOOR TREADMILLS

Almost every high street in every town has a gym with a treadmill, and whereas in the past runners had to train outdoors whatever the conditions, today treadmills offer the option of training indoors, with air conditioning and television screens replacing the wind, rain and countryside. My advice is to use treadmills as an occasional alternative only, with the bulk of marathon training outdoors. Biomechanically, treadmills differ from outdoor running and produce a slightly different running style, 'dragging' the leading leg back beneath the body rather than relying on the power of the leg to drive the body forwards. Scientific studies have found that the best way to counter this is to raise the treadmill to an incline of 1 per cent. Treadmill running also fails to replicate the variable gradients and terrain of running outdoors, and despite many of the distractions that gyms provide, running long distances on treadmills where the scenery never changes can be tedious and boring.

GPS

The thought of running while being monitored by a satellite in outer space was not one that entered the minds of marathon runners until recently, when portable Global Positioning Systems (GPS) were developed. GPS units not only monitor where a runner is, but how much distance they have covered, and the pace at which they are running. Since it is unlikely that anyone will ever get lost running in a well-organised marathon, the main

> **'Biomechanically, treadmills differ from outdoor running and produce a slightly different running style, 'dragging' the leading leg back beneath the body rather than relying on the power of the leg to drive the body forwards.'**

value of GPS is apparent during training, enabling runners to track and analyse their runs using computer software, and compare one run with another. In marathon races, mile and kilometre markers make it relatively easy to track distance covered and running speed, but when the going gets tough, and the course is not known, I have found that tracking each mile with GPS can really help, since it shows how much of each mile has been covered, and when the next mile marker should appear.

Marathons are not easy – if they were, everyone would run them. While many have run marathons without the support of any technology or science, using technological aids to complement rather than dominate training is a useful way of helping to prepare for the event.

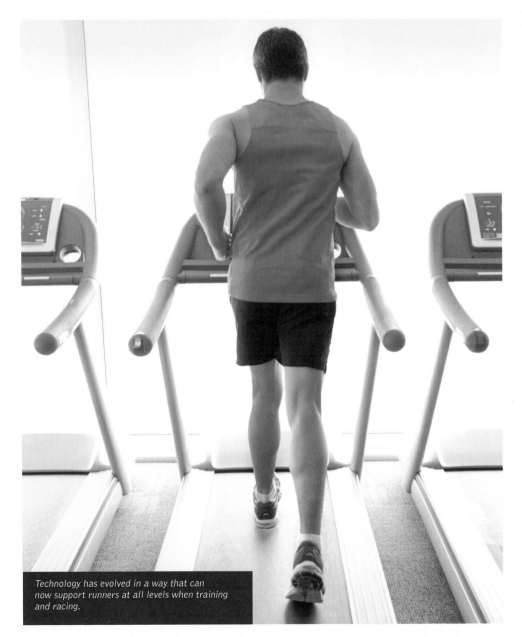

Technology has evolved in a way that can now support runners at all levels when training and racing.

RUNNING AT ALTITUDE

Sea-level marathons are hard work – go higher, where the air is thin, and the challenge of completing the distance is even harder.

One of the greatest pioneers of sport and exercise science, Griffith Pugh, conducted experiments supporting high-altitude expeditions climbing the Himalayas in the 1950s. He found what those who try to run at high altitude know only too well – that at heights of 2000m (6560ft) and above, the demands placed on the body increase inexorably, and running becomes significantly harder.

Around one-fifth of the air that runners breathe into their lungs at sea level consists of oxygen, which is vital for energy provision during marathons, and it may be a surprise to learn that this percentage remains the same as altitude increases – the problem is that the density of air gets progressively less as altitude increases, so there is less oxygen entering the lungs with each breath. The transport of oxygen from the lungs to the muscles also relies on air pressure, with oxygen under relatively high pressure entering the lungs, gradually moving down a 'pressure gradient' to the muscles. When air density is reduced at altitude, so too is pressure, and this makes the extraction of

> **'Athletes who do have to compete at altitude in endurance events such as marathons are normally advised to arrive at least one to two weeks in advance of their race to give time to adapt.'**

oxygen from air in the lungs more difficult, so less oxygen is supplied to the muscles.

The high-altitude environment is often referred to as being one that is 'hypoxic', or lacking in oxygen. To compensate, breathing frequency and heart rate both increase, which makes running feel much harder, and consequently performance will suffer. In 1968, Pugh used his Himalayan research to predict that endurance times at the Mexico Olympic Games, held at an

altitude of 2250m (7380ft), would suffer, and he was correct. Runners used to running at sea level struggled to get enough oxygen to their muscles, and either ran slower times, or suffered high levels of fatigue. Today, very few major marathons are held at locations higher than 2000m (6560ft), but scientists have found that with a period of acclimatisation, runners can adapt and cope with the high-altitude challenge. The main adaptation comes from an increase in the blood's concentration of haemoglobin, which can occur over 10–14 days. This is stimulated by the release of a hormone called

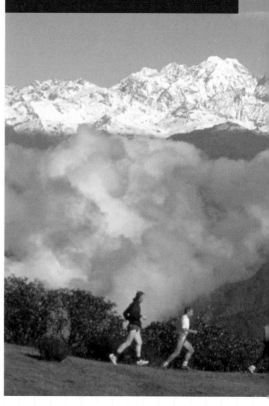

The thinner air and lower levels of oxygen at altitude can lead to changes that improve running performance at sea level.

erythropoietin, which has sadly gained notoriety as a means of illegally enhancing performance if injected rather than being produced naturally. Over time, heart and ventilation rates decrease, and running at altitude begins to feel similar to sea-level running.

Athletes who do have to compete at altitude in endurance events such as marathons are normally advised to arrive at least one to two weeks in advance of their race to give time to adapt. However, since scientific studies have shown that athletes who acclimatise to altitude are at an advantage when they return to sea level, many will use altitude training as part of their marathon preparation, wherever the event is to take place. The problem they face, though, is that during the first few days at altitude, the quality and quantity of training suffers, so current thinking involves a strategy of 'live high, train low'. This involves athletes sleeping and living at altitude, allowing the physiological adaptions to occur, but briefly returning to lower levels to train. There is also a risk that if haemoglobin levels become too high, the viscosity of the blood will increase, making it harder for blood and oxygen to penetrate deep into the muscles through the minute network of capillaries.

Altitude training and the associated adaptations largely remain part of the lifestyle of elite marathon runners, and not something that is on the radar of the majority of recreational runners. However, there are a few laboratories and commercial centres that offer runners the chance to train and adapt to hypoxic environments, as well as a number of marathons around the world over 2000m (6560ft) that runners of all abilities can enter.

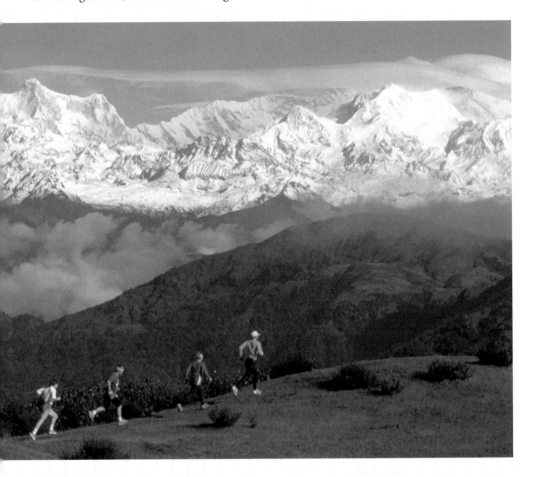

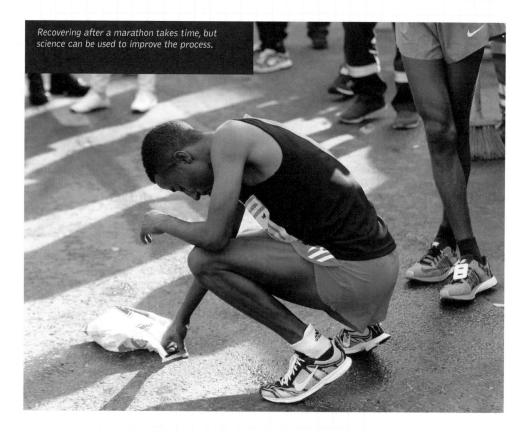

Recovering after a marathon takes time, but science can be used to improve the process.

THE SCIENCE OF RECOVERY

Using a science-based recovery strategy will help to optimise recovery after a run, and improve marathon training and racing performance.

Optimising recovery from training and racing is a crucial part of marathon success. When the hard work of running is over, the reduced physical demands of the recovery phase starts. The extent and duration of this period depends on the length and intensity of the run – after a short, hard session, warming down and removal of lactic acid from the blood and muscle are the main priority, whereas after a long endurance run, or after a marathon, replacing lost fluid and energy are critical.

Warming down is a technique that we explore further in Section Two (*see* page 104), but even after relatively short runs, fluid will be lost, and needs to be replaced. It is useful to get into the habit of weighing

yourself before and after a training session or race, since every 1kg (2.2lb) of weight lost is equivalent to around 1 litre (1¾ pints) of sweat that needs to be replaced as soon as possible, ideally with fluids that contain neither alcohol nor caffeine. Energy replacement is less critical after shorter runs, but carbohydrates still need to form the bulk of recovery meals, since regular failure to replace carbohydrate properly over days and weeks will gradually result in the depletion of glycogen stores and a build-up of fatigue.

When you cross the line at the end of a marathon, it is likely that even with on-course drinking, 2–4kg (4.4–8.8lb) of weight will have been lost, the majority of which will be as a result of fluid loss. This needs to be replaced quickly, and isotonic drinks, which also help to replace electrolytes, are effective in doing this. A crude but helpful indicator of post-race hydration status is urine colour – if it is dark, you are still dehydrated, whereas a light straw colour is a good indicator that a state of full hydration has been reached.

Running a marathon uses energy, and for recovery to be as quick and effective as possible, energy stores need to be replenished in a timely and efficient manner once the run has ceased. The total amount of energy expended running a marathon is around 3000 calories – equivalent to most male's daily food intake. This will have significantly depleted the body's stores of glycogen, and at the same time stimulated the activity of an enzyme called glycogen synthase, which is responsible for converting carbohydrates that have been eaten into glycogen in the muscle and liver. As a result, scientists have found that the first few hours after a run, when glycogen synthase is at its most active, provide a window of opportunity for rapid glycogen replacement if carbohydrate is eaten. However, fatigue

and physiological changes associated with marathon running often mean that runners don't feel like eating large quantities of food for some time after a race, so as a result energy drinks that are high in carbohydrate may be a useful substitution, while also helping with the process of rehydration.

Muscle fibres are damaged during a marathon by the relentless pounding and impacts from 35,000 strides. This will result in swelling, inflammation and ultimately pain, which normally peaks 48 hours after a marathon and lasts for a further 2–3 days. The use of massage and ice baths to possibly reduce this will be explored later in this book, but suffice it to say that for some, having sore legs and a strange walk is seen as a badge of honour that signals that a marathon has been completed!

Recovering from a marathon is relatively easy when compared with running one, and will happen with time regardless of whether or not a recovery plan is followed. However, with help and a recovery strategy, it is possible to enhance the recovery process after marathons and training, and ensure that you are prepared properly and effectively next time.

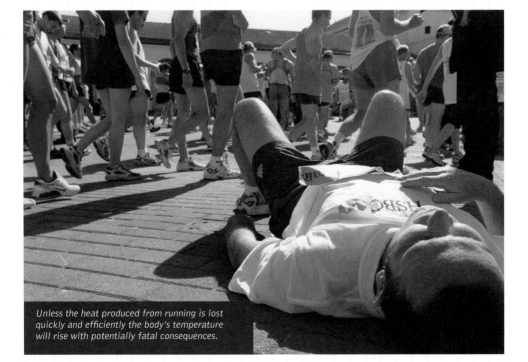

Unless the heat produced from running is lost quickly and efficiently the body's temperature will rise with potentially fatal consequences.

THERMOREGULATION – OR OVERHEATING

Marathon runners do not like it hot. Heat and humidity make it harder for them to keep cool, ensuring that long-distance running is an even greater challenge than normal.

At rest, our body temperature is around 37°C (99°F), but when running starts and the muscles contract, they also produce heat. As a result, body (or core) temperature starts to rise, until we are capable of losing heat at the same rate at which it is generated. At this point temperature plateaus at around 38–39°C (100–102°F). Sweating and the conduction of heat into the external environment are the body's main ways of losing heat, and ideally body temperature should remain in this 38–39°C (100–102°F) zone for the remainder of a training run or race.

However, when conditions are hot or humid (or both), it becomes much harder for runners to lose heat. Sweat 'drips' rather than evaporates, and with a lesser difference between skin temperature and the external environment, it is difficult for heat to transfer away from the body. Indeed, on really hot days there may even be heat transfer into

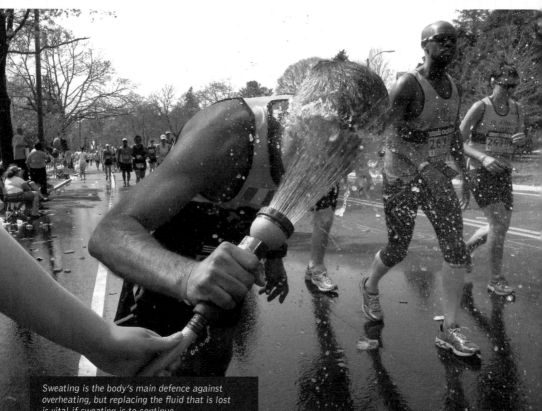

Sweating is the body's main defence against overheating, but replacing the fluid that is lost is vital if sweating is to continue.

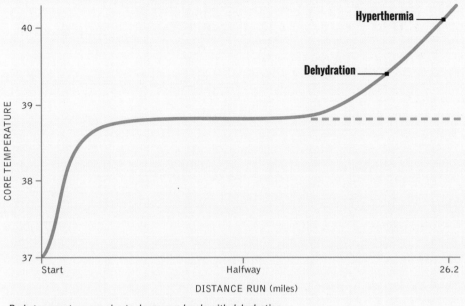

Body temperature can rise to dangerous levels with dehydration.

the body, rather than vice versa. This can make it really hard for the body to match heat loss with heat generation, and keep core temperature constant. When this no longer becomes possible, we see a second rise in core temperature, which if left unchecked can lead to potentially disastrous consequences.

When core temperature exceeds 40°C (104°F), a condition called hyperthermia is imminent. This is a situation in which the body is effectively overheating and normal functions start to suffer. Clear thinking becomes difficult, and runners lose coordination and start to fatigue rapidly. The heart has to work harder to divert more blood to the skin in an effort to cool down, and as a result less blood and oxygen reach the muscles and brain.

The body is faced with two options. The first, and most sensible, is to slow down so that less heat is produced and the equilibrium between heat production and heat loss is regained. In hot conditions, combining this with drinking fluids is important, since the fluids themselves help to cool the body, and crucially enable runners to continue sweating. The second option, which is more extreme, is for the body to adopt a

'When core temperature exceeds 40°C (104°F), a condition called hyperthermia is imminent. This is a situation in which the body is effectively overheating and normal functions start to suffer.'

horizontal position so that the supply of blood and oxygen to the brain is protected. This of course means lying down, which can occur consciously, or subconsciously through collapsing. I once ran a marathon on what proved to be one of the hottest days of the year, and it was an event described afterwards by an experienced runner as one that resembled a war zone rather than a race, with collapsed runners lying by the roadside along the course.

It is vital that marathon runners are aware of the additional challenge that they face on hot days, and are prepared to set more realistic goals and recognise the symptoms of overheating should they occur. Running marathons in hot conditions is possible, it just needs a rethink and refocus if the distance is to be completed safely and enjoyably. Most races start in the morning, so expect heat to rise as the race progresses, and if necessary slow down before your body tells you to stop!

THE BODY CLOCK

Some of us are morning runners, others prefer the evening. But when you can do nothing about a marathon start time, make sure you run well at the right time of day.

All of us are used to a pattern of waking and sleeping, a pattern that normally reflects the days' hours of daylight and darkness. While we are all aware of how we react and behave during these times, we are less conscious of a series of peaks and troughs that impact on areas such as alertness, body temperature, hunger and our readiness for exercise. This 24-hour pattern is governed by our circadian rhythm – basically an internal body clock driven by external factors such as daylight and darkness.

START TIMES

Plenty of scientists have investigated the impact of circadian rhythms on exercise and running, and found that the rhythms can impact on performance, depending on the time of day. It is not uncommon for some runners to feel sluggish in the morning, but more energetic later in the day. Others prefer to run earlier in the day, and struggle in the afternoon. Evidence suggests that most runners are at their 'physiological peak' towards the late afternoon or early evening, which lends physiological credence to undertaking training later in the day. However, I am not in favour of running too late in the evening, since this raises metabolic rate and body temperature at a time when the body should be shutting down and preparing for sleep.

Whatever your preference, the fact remains that the vast majority of marathons start in the morning, and runners must ensure that they are prepared for this. Unfortunately, many studies have found that

The body has a daily cycle of rhythms that help to control sleep and exercise, and aligning these with run times will improve performance.

first thing in the morning is not a good time for running – body temperature is low and it is unlikely that food will have been eaten for some time. I always advise runners to check the start time of their race some weeks in advance, and as race day approaches, begin to adjust their training times and body clock to the start time. Even the most committed of evening runners needs to get their body used to running at the same time as the race, otherwise standing on the start line on race day can be both a mental and psychological shock, and there is nothing worse than starting out on the 26.2-mile journey feeling sluggish from the outset. Getting used to an early start to the day, so that there is a time gap between waking and starting a run, also helps to set other bodily functions, including appetite and some that are more delicate – ensuring that your bowels are not full when the run or race starts!

TIME ZONES

Many runners of all abilities seek new challenges such as overseas marathons. When these mean crossing time zones, jet lag can be a problem, since the change in time disrupts the circadian rhythms. Scientists have found that the body adjusts to changes in time zone by between 60 and 90 minutes per day, with the adjustment seemingly taking longer after travel in an easterly direction. So if the time zone change is five hours, you should aim to arrive at least four to five days in advance to give your circadian rhythms a chance to reset. Researchers have found that early exposure to bright natural sunlight can help, and quickly resetting meal times, and exercising at the time of the race, will all enhance the adjustment process. The good news is that despite the undoubted feelings of tiredness that jet lag produces, studies have found that the impact on performance tends not to be too great.

Resetting your body clock so that it is used to running at the time when you need to run is important, ensuring that your training and preparation are optimised. This is more of a challenge with overseas races and time-zone changes, but by using simple techniques, you can still produce great performances at any time.

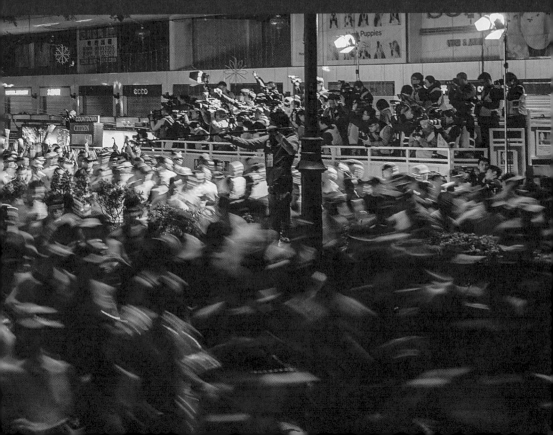

Marathon training can be tougher than running the race itself, but the use of science can help to make the journey to race day much easier.

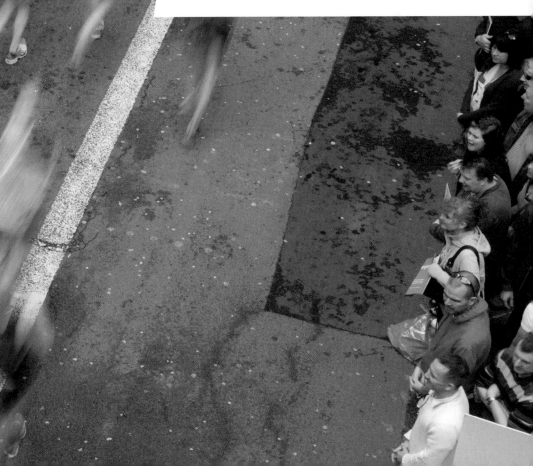

SECTION TWO
MARATHON TRAINING

From starting training to the week of the race, find out how to best apply sports science to prepare properly for the marathon.

STARTING OUT

It is often said that the hardest step of a marathon-training programme is the first one. But once underway, the journey has begun, and a marathon awaits.

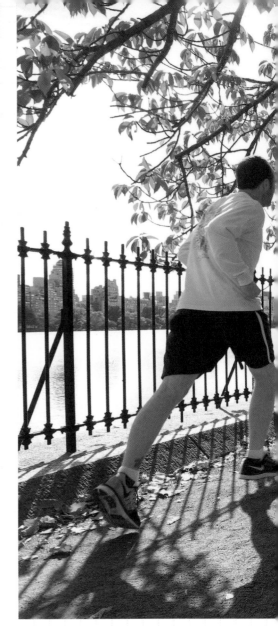

W hy would anyone want to put themselves through the training, dedication and pain that it takes to run 26.2 miles? There is no simple answer. In the past, marathons were competitive races for a hardy sub-group of serious runners. Today, they are mass-participation events, attracting runners of all shapes, sizes and abilities. Many are there for a once-only experience, just to be able to say they have run one. Others come back for more and many are driven by personal goals to raise charitable funds. It is also fair to say that quite a few runners find themselves on the start line by accident – a boast in front of friends and a subsequent race application with little expectation of getting a place – results in shock and desperation when the 'congratulations, you have been accepted' letter lands on the doormat a few weeks later.

So, where do you start on the quest to marathon success? Of course it depends on what level of fitness and running experience you have; if you are a serious couch potato, with little or no running and exercise background, asking your doctor for a health check is a sensible first step. Assuming all is well, the next stage is to invest in some sensible kit, with comfort and safety, not fashion, as the main priorities. A good running shop will help, and if the staff are good, they will be able to advise you on the type of footwear and running clothing that meet your needs. With many marathons held in the spring, training will take place during the darker winter nights, so seeing and being seen are important considerations.

At this stage, I always suggest that runners try to find a friend. Not one who enjoys going to the pub every night, but instead one who is also new to running, and perhaps even training for the same race. While you don't need to do every run together, having someone else at hand who is in the same situation and who can motivate you to train can be helpful over the long training months to come.

The next and very important stage is to start putting one foot in front of the other, even if the speed and duration are very slow to start with. Most runners learn that they have a marathon place five to six

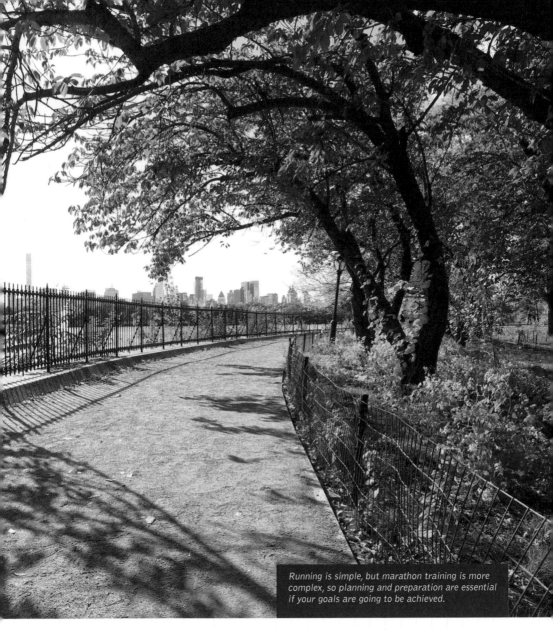

Running is simple, but marathon training is more complex, so planning and preparation are essential if your goals are going to be achieved.

months before race day, and this is ample time for even those with limited running or exercise experience to prepare. It also gives enough time to start out slowly and progress gradually, since trying to do too much too soon, and at too fast a pace, is one of the biggest mistakes made by many novices, and can soon lead to injury. At this early stage, it helps to have a realistic goal in mind, even if that needs to be changed at a later date. I always impress on marathon runners, and in particular first-timers, that

the number-one goal must be to complete the course, not compete with it. If it is your first marathon, it is highly unlikely that you will break the world record, and your expectations must be realistic.

Don't worry if your first training steps are walking – brisk walking is better than slow – your body will already be adapting and soon the walk will become a jog, your pace will increase, and you will find yourself running faster and for longer. The journey has begun!

TRAINING PRINCIPLES

Proper progression, a sensible intensity, and a strategic approach to race day combine to ensure that training is sensible, optimal and reduces the risk of injury.

The importance of specificity, progression, intensity and recovery was discussed in Section One (*see* pages 58–59). In practice, I always find that the best way to start planning a programme is to start at the end – the date of your marathon – then go back two weeks to allow for a period of tapering (when training load is reduced so that the body is ready for race day) and pre-race recovery, and work out how many training weeks you have to get ready. Once you have done this, don't panic! Just like

running a marathon, training for one is a slow and steady process, and you must pace yourself and not set off too quickly.

Running must, of course, form the main part of your training, and getting your body accustomed to running and being on your feet for a long period of time is fundamental to a training plan. If you are a novice, and training for your first marathon, you should initially aim to run for a period of time, not a set distance. If at first this is as little as 10–15 minutes, don't worry.

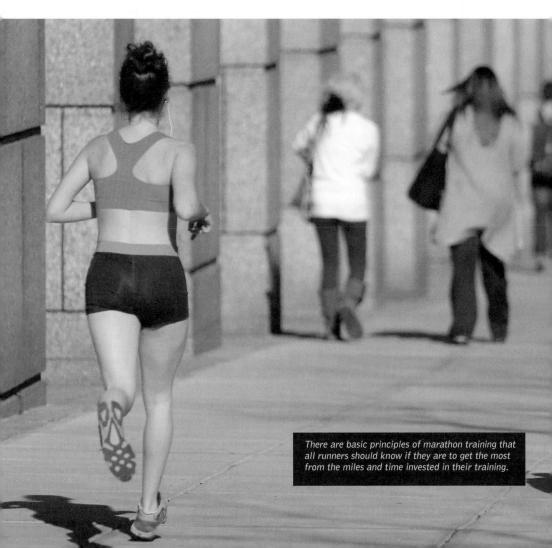

There are basic principles of marathon training that all runners should know if they are to get the most from the miles and time invested in their training.

MYTH: *MARATHON TRAINING IS BORING*

Doing too much of anything can become boring, so it's not surprising that running mile after mile to prepare for a marathon has the prospect of featuring high on a list of boring activities. Yet for many, running provides a way of de-stressing, and emptying the mind of the worries and issues of daily life, and with simple techniques even the longest of runs has the potential to pass quickly in a varied and even exciting manner.

Developing a portfolio of running routes, each with its own twists, turns and changes in scenery is the simplest way of adding variety, while simply running the same route in the opposite direction can make it seem surprisingly different. Running with a group, or with a friend, enables conversation and helps the miles to pass by, and when it comes to long distances, entering an organised race provides a competitive element, and even supporters, to help ease the coverage of each mile.

Many runners like to listen to music when running, while for many others, running is a time when the mind can be cleared, and problems tackled and solved with no interruptions. Visualising rewarding or enjoyable situations, such as finishing the marathon you are training for, is also a great way of distracting from the miles. Using these techniques can transform running from a tedious experience to one that can be therapeutic and even relaxing, and as the months of training unfold and the seasons change, the same route can easily look remarkably different.

'Don't be surprised if you initially put on some weight – it takes a long time to lose body fat, but a lot less time to gain muscle, so as your muscles become stronger, you may well see your weight increase slightly.'

With every session your body is responding to the stimulus of training, and adapting by improving your oxygen-transport system, as well as strengthening the muscles, tendons and ligaments that support each stride. Don't be surprised if you initially put on some weight – it takes a long time to lose body fat, but a lot less time to gain muscle, so as your muscles become stronger, you may well see your weight increase slightly.

Very quickly, a run that felt hard when your training commenced will start to feel much easier. This is the time to start progressing, at first by increasing the duration of your run, then running speed. At the outset, it will take quite a while to recover after a run – at least a day or so. This is because of the stress that the muscle fibres have been put under, and as they recover and repair, there will be some soreness that will take a while to disappear. Don't worry about taking time off – in fact it is essential to do so, since trying to do too much too soon, and not giving time to recover and adapt, increases the risk of injury.

As we will explore later, the most important run of the training week is the 'long run', which most runners find easiest to perform at the weekend. An anecdotal method for developing the long run is to increase its length by no more than 10 per cent per week. Most runners, scientists and coaches advocate that there should be at least one long run of 20–22 miles included into a marathon-training plan, which should be two to three weeks before the race itself. This is where working backwards from race day can really help, so you can calculate what your longest run should be on the weeks leading up to the race, and – importantly – ensures that you don't overload your body too quickly.

There are plenty of marathon-training programmes available for runners, and we have included some on pages 176–179. Training for a marathon is not an exact science, and there are many different ways of preparing for the big event. There is no harm in occasionally training in a format other than running – cycling or swimming for example – but these alternatives should be used exceptionally, not regularly. There comes a point when finding additional time for training becomes difficult, if not impossible. This is when you should consider increasing intensity, either by running the distance more quickly, or running a series of fast and slow bursts within the run.

Adhering to the primary principles of training is vital during marathon training and ensures that you progress at the right speed and intensity, minimising the risk of injury and ensuring that you peak at the right time.

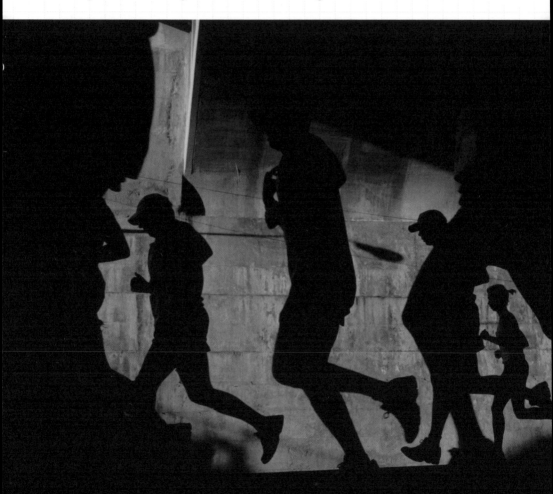

Each step of your training plays a small part in making the physical and mental changes your body needs so that you can run 26.2 miles.

MYTH: *IF I GET INJURED OR ILL I WILL HAVE TO WITHDRAW FROM MY MARATHON*

Of course no one wants to lose training time as a result of injury or illness, but these are both occupational hazards of marathon training. The closer an illness or injury occurs to race day, the bigger the problem, and if medical advice is clear that running a marathon is not possible, then withdrawal is the only option. Many major marathons allow runners who withdraw to defer their entry for 12 months, alleviating some of the inevitable disappointment.

If it is just a couple of weeks of running that fall by the wayside during the early or middle stages of the training programme, then don't despair. It is relatively easy to make up for lost time and mileage, although it is important to ease back into running gradually, rather than trying to restart with the same intensity

and volume that was manageable before the injury or illness occurred. However, when the enforced lay-off is longer, and crucial weeks of training towards the end of a programme have been scuppered, resetting of race-day targets and goals is an option, provided that you are fit to run. Completing a marathon does not, after all, need to involve running at a fast speed or intensity – with a combination of slow running, and even walking, it is still possible to cover 26.2 miles in a reasonable time and well within the cut-off for most marathons.

Deciding whether to withdraw or to race after illness or injury is a difficult and sometimes very personal decision, but if you are well enough to run, and prepared to accept a slower finish time, completion is still possible.

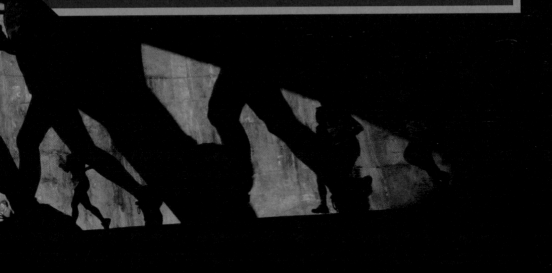

ASSESSING YOUR FITNESS AND RUNNING STYLE

Once the domain of elite runners, laboratories now offer to assess the fitness and style of runners from all backgrounds. But does a lab test work, and offer worthwhile performance enhancement?

Beginning the long journey towards a marathon medal is often the hardest part of a training programme, and knowing where you are at the outset, and fine tuning your training and running style so that you optimise your running and reduce the risk of injury, can prove to be a worthwhile investment for many.

Advances in exercise physiology mean that we can now accurately assess a runner's level of fitness, and the optimal speed for different parts of the training programme. Similar developments in biomechanics and motion analysis mean that we can look at running technique and determine what might need to be changed. Just a few years ago these types of assessment were only offered to elite athletes, but today many universities and commercial centres offer

runners of all abilities the chance to gain a greater insight into their personal physiology and running style.

But is it worth it, and what does it tell you? A runner who visits a sports science laboratory for a physiological assessment is likely to face a series of tests and measures that will include their body fat percentage to determine their optimum weight (if you weigh too much extra energy will be needed in training and racing). They will almost certainly also undergo measurements of their heart rate and oxygen uptake over a series of progressively increasing running speeds, culminating in maximum effort to determine their maximum oxygen uptake and heart rate. At the same time, measures of lactic acid may be taken to find the running speed at which this starts to increase. All of these figures can

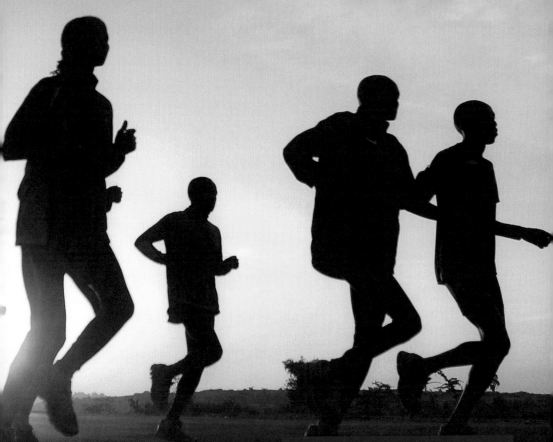

Optimising the time spent training ensures that your body adapts steadily and specifically to the demands of running a marathon.

be combined to build a picture of a runner's current level of fitness, and to guide and fine-tune their running speeds in training.

One drawback, though, is that this is a simple 'snapshot' in time, and the measures could soon change in a positive way after a period of training, or regress after injury or illness. Regular testing helps to monitor progress over time, but all of this comes at a significant cost, and runners need to weigh this against the gains that are made. While this sort of knowledge can be very helpful to both athletes and coaches, it is worth bearing in mind that there are many runners who have trained for, and completed marathons, without ever having had any form of physiological assessment.

Analysis of running style has also become available to runners from all backgrounds, and can range from basic filming while on a treadmill, to more complex three-dimensional assessment of movement patterns and forces. An assessment of this nature can help a runner to iron out any movements or habits that expend extra energy and make running less efficient. It can also be used to identify the type of running shoe that suits a particular running style, and as a consequence reduce the risk of injury. However, as discussed on page 42, there are many occasions when a runner may look ungainly, yet have a running style that suits them and their biomechanics. Care also needs to be taken when interpreting information from individuals who may not be used to running on treadmills, since this action in itself can have a short-term impact on the way a runner runs.

DIFFERENT TRAINING APPROACHES

Marathon training is not easy, but not every approach entails a radical lifestyle change. Sacrifices must be made, and core elements such as a long weekly run are key to success.

Training for a marathon is not an exact science, and there are many different ways of preparing your body to run 26.2 miles. Which method you decide to follow depends on many factors, including your experience, goals and – crucially – your lifestyle. Most coaching manuals recommend a complete change in your daily habits, sacrificing family time and recreation for hours and miles of training. This is one approach, and there is no doubt that it is effective, but there are others that will work too, reflecting the fine balance between training load, time, injury prevention and of course, success.

Marathon-training programmes normally recommend five or six days of training per week, with one or two days for recovery. This is an ideal scenario, giving every chance of developing the leg strength and cardiovascular endurance that a marathon requires. At the other extreme, I have a running partner who regularly completes marathons in around 4 hours, but these are based on just one training session per week. While this defies all the marathon-coaching manuals, the 'once' and 'six a week' methods have one thing in common – the weekly long run. This is the most important component of any marathon-training programme. There is little benefit in training for six days per week if your longest run never exceeds 6 miles, but you can accomplish a marathon if you only train once a week, so long as this single session is a gradually progressing long run that reaches a distance in excess of 20 miles.

Of course this single-run-a-week approach is never going to produce a tremendous time, but it is possible to use it and successfully complete the distance. It can be attractive to those who have busy lifestyles filled with work, commuting and family commitments, but it won't develop the endurance and strength that comes from more training days and more miles.

The long run is important from both a physiological and psychological perspective and due to time constraints, most runners will include it within their training at the weekend. It conditions the body to run with low muscle-glycogen stores, while developing the mental resilience

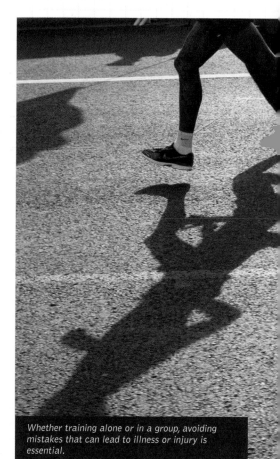

Whether training alone or in a group, avoiding mistakes that can lead to illness or injury is essential.

and confidence that are needed to run marathons. There are no hard and fast rules about exactly how far your longest run should be, but one run of at least 20 miles should be the minimum that you aim for. At the same time, progression towards this longest run should include a series of runs over slightly shorter distances – 16, 17, 18 and 19 miles – it is these that will develop the physiological adaptations that are needed, while runs over 20 miles will have a crucial psychological benefit. In an ideal world, your training should include runs that approach 26 miles. This is normal for elites, who have the time and conditioning to support this method. In reality, for many of us this is not possible, so it is critical that your training lays the foundations upon which the final race-day push to 26.2 miles can be made.

The weekly long run challenges the body to run with low glycogen stores, but science has shown that this can also be achieved with back to back shorter runs. If a run of 12–15 miles is followed by a low-carbohydrate diet, you can begin your run the next day with low glycogen stores. This is certainly not recommended for racing, but it means you only need to be 6–8 miles into the second run before you begin to replicate the low glycogen conditions that occur 18–20 miles into a marathon, making back-to-back runs a simpler and more attractive alternative to a single long run.

Don't be put off by those who say your lifestyle has to change radically to run a marathon. Of course it is not easy, and sacrifices will need to be made however you decide to train. Your longest run is critical, alongside a sensible and realistic race-day target time and strategy.

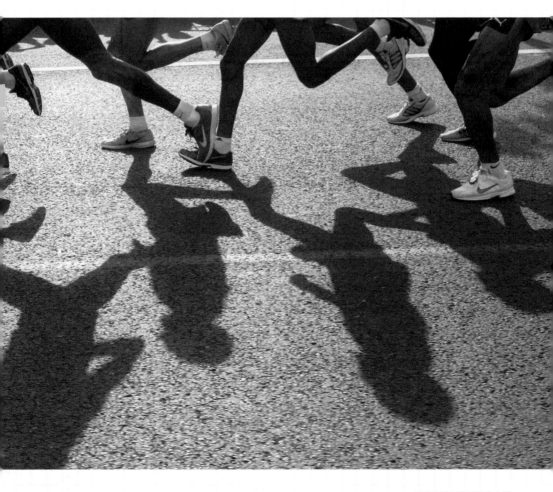

COACHING AND RUNNING WITH OTHERS

Finding a friend or coach to motivate, mentor or train with can make the long hard months of marathon training much easier, and more effective.

Before the growth of mass-participation marathons, the only people completing the distance were serious – and in some cases fanatical – runners whose lives were dedicated to running, and for whom the pain and discomfort of training was second nature. They invariably belonged to running clubs where there were plenty of other like-minded runners, entered races regularly, and had access to a coach. In the pre-internet days of communication, face-to-face contact was crucial for all-important advice, training plans and coaching.

Today, joining a club can be daunting, but most modern running clubs will cater for runners of all abilities. Regular club training nights – normally two per week – provide an opportunity to train with others and the motivation to run when your instincts are telling you to remain indoors. There are normally club runs at the weekend as well, frequently over increasingly long distances as major marathons approach, helping to make running feel easier and more sociable.

One of the best ways to stay motivated and focussed on your training is to follow a training plan. On pages 176–179 of this book I have produced marathon-training plans that reflect different lifestyles and abilities, and there are many other similar programmes

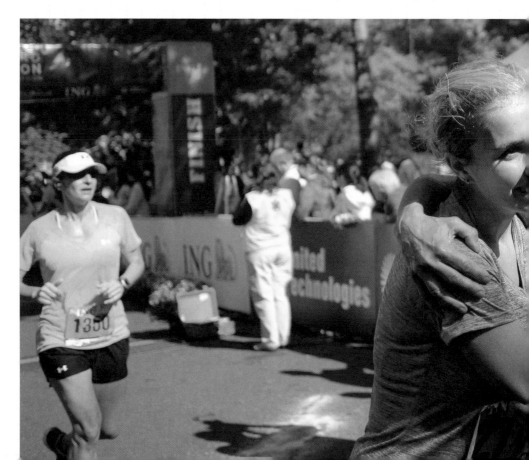

accessible on the internet or published in running magazines. They will all work – while science can enhance training and performance, it is not an exact art form, and there are many different ways to reach the same successful endpoint. If you prefer not to join a club but still want to receive coaching, personal coaching support can be obtained through the internet. Here, training plans are personalised and updated regularly by your coach, and there may also be an opportunity for personal communication. However, this will come at a cost, dependent on the level of service that is required.

Once you have a programme, whether a general one, or one from an internet or club coach, running with a friend can be very motivational, and you can help each other to run at times when things are getting tough. However, it is important to select your running partner carefully, since as we have discussed, running at the correct intensity is an important prerequisite for marathon-training success. Waking up on a weekend morning faced with the prospect of a long

and lonely run is not everyone's idea of the best start to a day, but knowing that there is a friend or club mates who can cover the same distance with you, at an intensity that suits your needs, can help enormously.

A note of caution – you need to ensure that you don't get carried away by the enthusiasm of others, and attempt more than you are capable of. This is especially true for novice marathon runners, whose needs may not always be reflected in the demands and programmes from some coaches, who may be more used to training and helping experienced runners for whom a finishing time is more important than a marathon completion.

Having someone to support your marathon training, both in terms of advice and running company, can help to get you through the months of preparation. But as your confidence and fitness grow, it is important to motivate yourself and take responsibility for your own training and fitness, ensuring that you train in a manner that suits you.

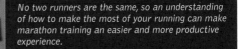

No two runners are the same, so an understanding of how to make the most of your running can make marathon training an easier and more productive experience.

SETTING AN ACHIEVABLE TARGET TIME

Most runners have an ideal target time for their marathon. To ensure this time is based on fact and science, not fiction, this chart indicates the running pace that is needed to achieve a range of finishing times.

The chart also shows the intermediate times that are needed for distances between the start to the finish, so that a proper and realistic pacing strategy can be developed. But be warned – if your target time results in a running pace that is faster than that achieved in your pre-marathon training and racing, you won't sustain this pace for 26.2 miles, so be realistic, and reset your goal.

RUNNING PACE CHART

min/ mile pace	5 miles	10 miles	13.1 miles	15 miles	20 miles	25 miles	26.2 miles
15	1 hr 15 min	2 hr 30 min	3 hr 17 min	3 hr 45 min	5 hr	6 hr 15 min	6 hr 33 min
12	60 min	2 hr	2 hr 37 min	3 hr	4 hr	5 hr	5 hr 14 min
10	50 min	1 hr 40 min	2 hr 11 min	2 hr 30 min	3 hr 20 min	4 hr 10 min	4 hr 22 min
9	45 min	1 hr 30 min	1 hr 58 min	2 hr 15 min	3 hr	3 hr 45 min	3 hr 56 min
8	40 min	1 hr 20 min	1 hr 45 min	2 hr	2 hr 40 min	3 hr 20 min	3 hr 30 min
7	35 min	1 hr 10 min	1 hr 32 min	1 hr 55 min	2 hr 20 min	2 hr 55 min	3 hr 03 min
6	30 min	60 min	1 hr 19 min	1 hr 30 min	2 hr	2 hr 30 min	2 hr 37 min
5	25 min	50 min	1 hr 06 min	1 hr 15 min	1 hr 40 min	2 hr 05 min	2 hr 11 min

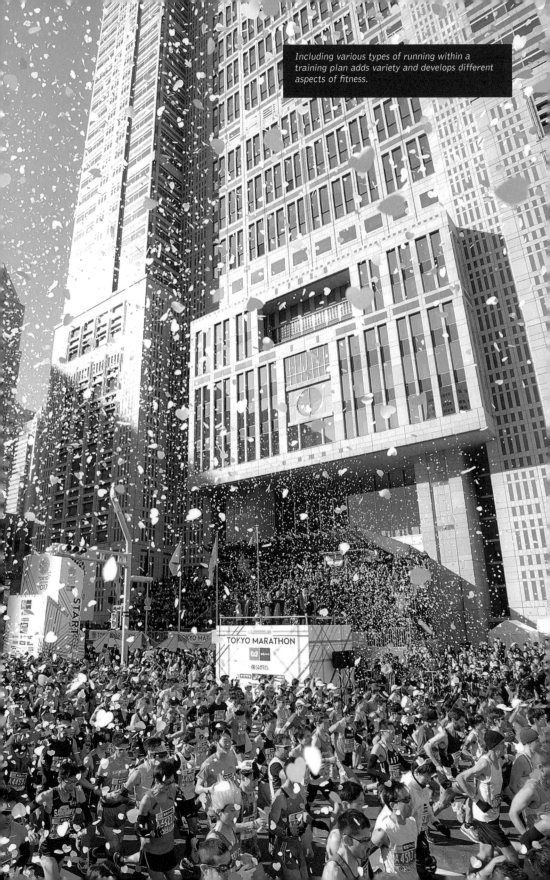

Including various types of running within a training plan adds variety and develops different aspects of fitness.

When you stand on the start line, you must have a sensible time in mind that is based on your previous training and racing performances.

MYTH: *IF I CAN RUN 20 MILES, I CAN RUN A MARATHON*

When training for a marathon, the importance of the weekly long run cannot be underestimated, and as a result, most training programmes focus on a run of at least 20 miles before tackling the marathon's 26.2 miles. But achieving 20 miles is no guarantee of success – the remaining 6.2 miles is 31 per cent further than 20 miles, and many experienced runners would argue that they require a lot more than 31 per cent of extra effort! Moreover, attempting to run 26.2 miles at the same pace you used for the 20-mile run is almost certainly going to lead to disaster over the last few miles.

Being capable of running 20 miles once is not an indicator of marathon success. The number of runs at distances between 16 and 20 miles is also important, since it is the combination of these, rather than a single one-off long run, that leads to physiological adaptations that develop endurance. That said, if you can run 20 miles, then barring disaster, you should be capable of completing a marathon. The last few miles will be hard, and unless the 20-mile run is one of many over a similar distance, the remaining 6.2 will only be possible with a sensible pacing strategy.

Completing a 20-mile training run should be one part of a successful marathon strategy, and ideally it will be part of a series of runs of similar length, if not longer. If 22–24 miles can be achieved in training, the mental and physical challenge of 26.2 miles will become just a little bit easier.

MYTH: *IF I RUN A MARATHON I WILL LOSE LOTS OF WEIGHT*

It is true that by the time you have run 26.2 miles, your weight will be significantly less than it was on the start line. But much of that decrease will have come from a loss of fluid, mainly in the form of sweat, which could easily account for 3 or 4 kilograms of weight. This will soon be put back on once you start to drink and rehydrate after the race. Long term weight loss comes from a loss of body fat, which is stored in various sites around the body, and it is all too easy to hope that these stores will have reduced or even disappeared after a marathon has been run. However, each gram of body fat contains 9 calories of energy and the average energy cost of running a marathon is around 3000 calories. This is equivalent to just 330 grams of body fat, so any large-scale weight loss after a marathon will just be temporary, and sadly the long-term loss of body fat is much less than many runners imagine. Runners need to run around 80 miles to use the energy contained in just 1 kilogram of body fat, but using marathon training and running as a means of losing weight is not recommended. Marathon runners must refuel and replace energy efficiently, otherwise the deficit in energy intake that results from training and trying to lose weight will simply result in extra fatigue, illness or even injury.

DESIGNING A TRAINING PROGRAMME

There are many ways to train for a marathon. Not all are the same, yet most will work. Choosing what is best for you can make a huge difference to your success on race day.

The goal of any marathon-training programme, whether it is for an elite athlete or a marathon first-timer, is quite simple: it is to condition the human body to complete 26.2 miles as efficiently and quickly as possible. For some, this means developing the ability to run at speeds close to 13 miles per hour for 2 hours, for others it is simply to complete the distance.

No two marathon-training programmes are the same, and from the outset they need to reflect the running experience, marathon experience, and fitness of a runner. A programme must also be pragmatic – the vast majority of marathon runners on the start line have day jobs and families,

> **'Weekly recovery days are also vital, giving the body time to adapt to the stimulus of training, but so too is the taper period that lasts for the two weeks before the marathon.'**

and cannot devote the same time to their training that elite runners do. Time and again, I have seen and spoken with novice marathon runners who have been scared by programmes that come close to replicating the weekly mileage and lifestyle of elites, suggesting that this is the only way to train for a marathon. It is not – in fact it is almost certainly the wrong way, since doing too much can easily lead to fatigue and almost certain injury in runners who have not spent years conditioning their bodies to the rigours of intensive training.

As we will explore further later on, regardless of the training programme you have followed, your race-day target time and strategy are critical – I have seen the most intensive programmes that have delivered well-trained runners undone by a mindless approach to race day, whereas programmes

that may not on the face of it seem to be ideal can still deliver marathon success with a sensible approach to the race.

In Section One (*see* pages 58–59), we discussed the main scientific principles of marathon training – progression, overload, recovery and specificity. These of course need to be borne in mind when following a programme, and should be reflected by a gradual increase in total mileage, running intensity, and the length of the all-important weekly long run. Weekly recovery days are also vital, giving the body time to adapt to the stimulus of training, but so too is the taper period that lasts for the two weeks before the marathon.

In my view, experienced runners used to running a distance of 10–13 miles should

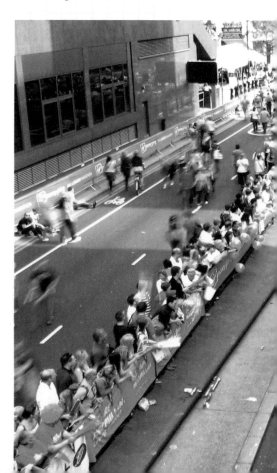

Weeks to go	16	15	14	13	12	11	10	9	8	7	6	5	4	3	2	1	Race day
Longest run (in miles)	10	11	12	13	14	15	16	17	18	19	20	21	22	22	13	10	26.2

be comfortably capable of training for, and running, a marathon. My rule of thumb is that to be ready for a spring marathon, a runner should be able to run 10 miles by the start of the year. This should allow close to four months of training to develop a solid aerobic base and leg strength, and to gradually extend the weekly long run from 10 miles to 20–22 miles. It also allows for inevitable periods of illness or injury when training may have to be put on hold. Increasing the long-run length by 1 mile per week is a sensible aim, and should ensure that with a month or more to go before race day, the 20–22-mile distance has been accomplished.

Runners with less experience, or who are complete novices, should try to start earlier, and may well need an extra two months of progressively increasing mileage to adapt their bodies. At its simplest level, I find it can really help to chart marathon-training progress by the distance of the longest run, as the simple chart above shows.

If a runner can keep to these targets, there is no doubt that they will be able to complete a marathon, no matter how many other training sessions are included between each long run. Additional sessions will improve both the quality of training, and running speed, making the last few miles seem much easier. Training for, and running a marathon is all about balancing a lifetime goal with a lifestyle choice.

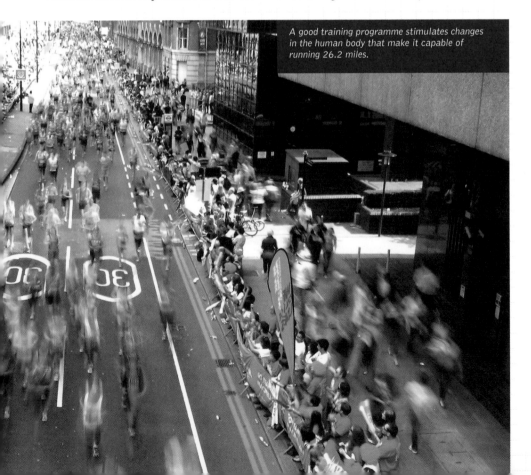

A good training programme stimulates changes in the human body that make it capable of running 26.2 miles.

TRAINING ZONES AND HEART RATE MONITORS

Using heart rate to fine tune training so that it is neither too tough nor too easy can be tricky, but is made simpler by understanding how to use a heart rate monitor properly.

We have already established that running at the right speed – or intensity – is a crucial part of a successful training programme, and of course this also has an impact on the target time for race day. While continually training at a high intensity risks burn-out and injury, if intensity is too low, it simply won't overload the body's systems to a level that results in adaptations and improvements. Furthermore, targeting a time for the 26.2 miles that represents a pace that you have never comfortably achieved in training is both unrealistic and a recipe for disaster on race day.

The secret to success is a mixture of intensities that provide variety to your running, while developing aerobic capacity and endurance. Since the body's ability to sustain a high exercise intensity decreases proportionally with the distance run, it follows that shorter runs can be run at a high intensity, with longer runs at a lower intensity. This doesn't mean that all short runs have to be at a high intensity, since recovery is vital, and running short distances at a low intensity should form part of a recovery strategy while still adding miles to your training.

It is also possible to incorporate low- and

Today's runners are able to use technology to enhance performance in a way that was never possible in the past.

high-intensity training into the same session. One common way of doing this is by fartlek running, a technique that originated in Scandinavia. It involves alternating bursts of high- and low-intensity running, based on how you feel during a run. A more structured approach to achieving the same objective is interval running, where the alternating intensities are set by either time or distance.

A general principle is that high-intensity running develops the cardiovascular system and aerobic capacity, whereas lower-intensity running develops the strength and endurance in the legs that is needed to run a marathon. Both are needed, since an improved aerobic capacity makes running feel easier, and as we found in Section One (*see* page 28), running at a lower relative exercise intensity places much less physiological and metabolic strain on the body.

Some runners like to use heart rate monitors to help judge the intensity of their training. They should be seen as an aid, not an obsession. Studies investigating the link between heart rate and training intensity have produced the chart below, which shows – approximately – the training zone related to each heart rate.

Scientists have found that one of the most effective training intensities for the development of oxygen-uptake capacity is to run at a speed just below that where lactic acid starts to rise rapidly. This is often called 'tempo' running, and normally equates to a heart rate of around 80 per cent maximum. As a marathon-training programme progresses, the split between low, moderate and high-intensity exercise can change. At the outset, I would expect to see a ratio of 70:20:10 when it comes to sessions involving low, medium and high-intensity running, shifting to 50:30:20 as the race approaches. This allows for a gradual development of mileage and distance, while including high-intensity running for aerobic capacity.

With experience, it should become possible to listen to and understand your body without the need for heart rate monitors and technology. But with or without technology, using a simple blend of distance and varying intensity is crucial for the development of marathon fitness.

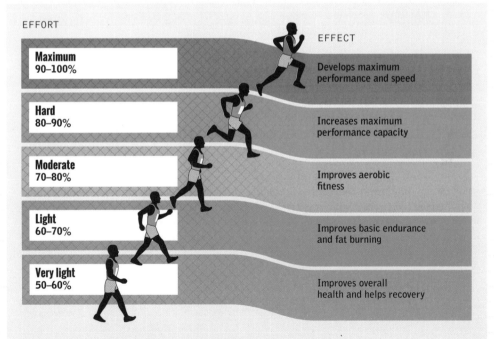

EFFORT

EFFECT

Maximum
90–100%

Develops maximum performance and speed

Hard
80–90%

Increases maximum performance capacity

Moderate
70–80%

Improves aerobic fitness

Light
60–70%

Improves basic endurance and fat burning

Very light
50–60%

Improves overall health and helps recovery

Heart rate zones can be used to fine-tune training intensity.

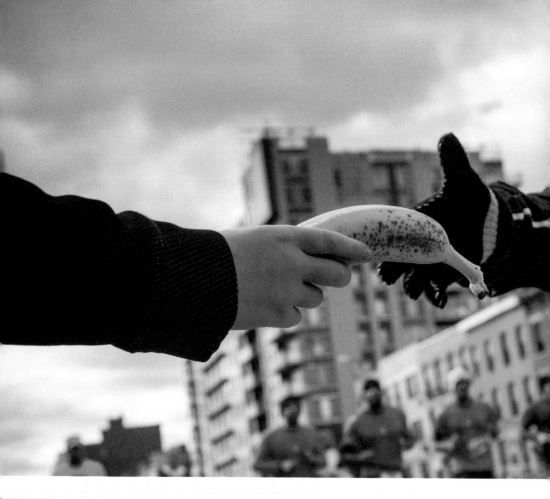

TRAINING NUTRITION

Without the right fuel, performance will suffer, and it's not just about race day. Supporting training with nutrition is just as important as eating the right foods just before and on the big day.

The human body, and especially that of someone training to run a marathon, requires good-quality food if it is to function at its best. As we have seen, performances in training, including the capacity to train at the right intensity and to recover afterwards, are crucial if your preparations for a marathon are going to go well, so focussing on correct nutrition in the months and weeks before a marathon is just as important as the last few days before the race.

Our diets consist of three main macronutrients: fat, protein and carbohydrate. Fat is very energy dense, containing lots of calories, but unfortunately not the sort that provide energy at the rate needed for marathon running. Protein helps to repair damaged tissues and provide the building blocks for the body, but only has limited value as an energy provider. On the other hand, carbohydrate is vital for energy, since it is converted into glycogen once eaten and stored in the liver and muscle as the main fuel for running.

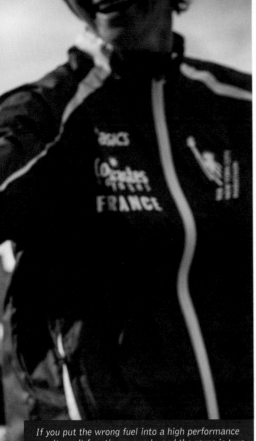

If you put the wrong fuel into a high performance car, it won't function properly, and the same is true for the human body.

Knowing the key role of carbohydrate for marathon runners, and the importance of early refuelling to capitalise on the heightened activity of glycogen synthase, the enzyme responsible for converting carbohydrate to glycogen, it is easy to understand the value of a daily high-carbohydrate diet in training. At the same time, it is important to be sensible, since eating too much of any food can cause weight to increase, if energy intake exceeds energy expenditure. A 6-mile run is likely to use around 700 calories for most people, so this needs to be factored in when judging the food quantities used for refuelling.

The supply of nutritional supplements for sports people has become a massive business, but I always recommend that 'food comes first', since there is no substitute for a good high-carbohydrate diet. Supplements can contain a range of ingredients, from carbohydrate to caffeine, and from amino acids to vitamins. As long as you have a good diet, a lot of money can be saved from not purchasing supplements. When coaching celebrity runners, I always emphasise the importance of diet to support training, but occasionally suggest

'A 6-mile run is likely to use around 700 calories for most people, so this needs to be factored in when judging the food quantities used for refuelling.'

Since our glycogen stores are sufficient to fuel most runs up to a distance of around 18 miles, the majority of marathon-training runs, especially during the early stages of a programme, will not face an energy crisis due to a loss of glycogen – it is only when a run is longer than 18 miles that this can become an issue. That said, shorter runs over consecutive days can present a cumulative energy problem if sufficient carbohydrate is not eaten. A 6-mile run will use around one-third of available glycogen, so this will not impact on performance, but if stores are not refuelled properly afterwards, the next run will eat into energy stores further still. If this continues over days or even weeks, poor nutrition will lead to a gradual decrease in glycogen causing even the shortest of runs to feel hard and training to suffer.

a daily multivitamin with iron, simply for 'insurance', especially as race day gets closer. Iron is important since it is needed for the production of haemoglobin, the part of the blood that carries oxygen from the lungs to the muscles, which if low can result in a condition called anaemia. This can be a problem for all runners, but particularly so for females at specific times of their monthly cycle.

Nutrition provides fuel, and fuel is needed for energy. Supporting training and racing with the right nutritional strategy is therefore crucial for marathon success and sustained high-quality training and racing performances.

TRAINING HYDRATION

Your body loses fluid when running and, if left unchecked, dehydration and a drop in performance soon occur. Supporting training with hydration is an essential task for all marathon runners.

Alongside a loss of fuel, the second key challenge faced by marathon runners is the loss of fluid, which mainly arises as a consequence of the need to stay cool, and prevent core body temperature rising to dangerous levels. Provided that the pre-run diet is high in carbohydrate, we have seen that fuel loss only becomes critical during the latter stage of a long run. But a runner's hydration status, which reflects levels of body fluid, becomes critical at a much earlier stage during both training and running a marathon, particularly in hot and humid conditions.

In Section One we explored the science behind sweating and fluid loss, and the importance of allowing sweat to evaporate from the skin so that heat created by running is lost. This occurs in training as well as in marathons, and often at a rate that could be as high as 2–3 litres (3½– 5¼ pints) per hour. We know that sweat loss (or dehydration) exceeding 2 per cent of bodyweight is detrimental to physical and mental performance, and for a runner weighing 75kg (11st 8lb, or 165lb), this equates to just 1.5 litres (2½ pints) of sweat. This could arise in less than an hour, particularly if conditions are warm, and the run is at a high intensity. Dehydration can occur at the same rate in both a marathon and a training run, but organised marathons normally take account of the need to replace lost fluid, and provide drink stations on the route. The London Marathon, for example, has water stations every mile between miles 3 and 25, as well as isotonic drinks at 5, 10, 15, 19 and 23 miles. Training runs, of course, seldom have drink stations, yet their duration and distances can quickly result in sweat loss that exceeds the 2 per cent performance threshold.

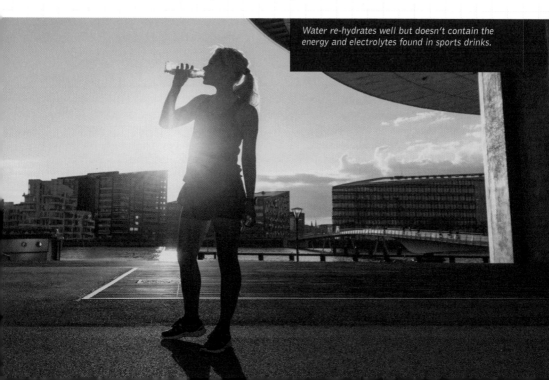

Water re-hydrates well but doesn't contain the energy and electrolytes found in sports drinks.

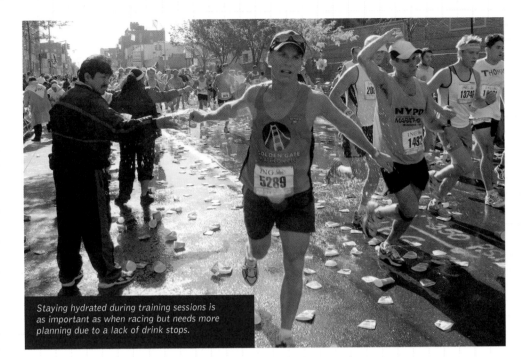

Staying hydrated during training sessions is as important as when racing but needs more planning due to a lack of drink stops.

There are some simple, practical steps that runners can take to combat dehydration during training. The first is to ensure that you are properly hydrated before starting your run, and the best way to do this is by checking the colour of your urine; ideally it should be pale yellow in colour – too dark, and you are dehydrated. The second is to take fluid with you, especially on runs longer than 5 or 6 miles. Some runners will carry bottles of fluid that are shaped to fit into the hand, while on longer runs some will run with camel packs – lightweight back packs filled with fluid, with a tube to the mouth for frequent drinking. Another option I like to use is to store a drink on your running route, which works particularly well if you are running laps, so that fluid is provided at regular intervals. Finally, it is important to replace fluids lost when training as soon as the run is over – each 1kg (2.2lb) of weight loss equates to 1 litre (1¾ pints) of fluid, so weighing yourself before and after a run shows how much fluid needs to be replaced.

In Section One on pages 38–39, we explored the science behind hydration, and outlined the efficient way in which isotonic drinks can replace fluid, energy and electrolytes. Because isotonic drinks are absorbed quickly, they are normally the best type of drink to consume while running, especially when the run is long, and energy loss is a challenge. During and after runs that are less than 13 or 14 miles in length, when loss of energy is less likely to be an issue, water is a very effective and simple way of rehydrating, although the need to replace energy that has been used after the run remains important, which is where isotonic drinks, or carbohydrate foods, have a role to play. Other drinks such as milk, chocolate milk and even coconut water have gained popularity in recent years. Milk-based drinks contain a blend of carbohydrate and protein, and as a result are better used for post-run recovery. Coconut water is similar to many commercial isotonic drinks, containing carbohydrate, electrolytes and fluid and provides an alternative means of hydrating and refuelling.

Good hydration is, then, just as important for training as it is for running marathons. It is a challenge faced by runners at an earlier stage, and over shorter distances, than the energy challenge, so must not be overlooked.

WARMING UP AND WARMING DOWN

Warming up and warming down, terms given to the immediate preparation phases before and after a run, are tasks that most runners know they need to do, but not necessarily with an awareness of why they need to do them.

The rationale for each is different. When it comes to warming up, as we saw in Section One on pages 22–23, the biochemical reactions needed to produce energy within the muscle are complex, and as any chemistry teacher will tell you, a reaction occurs more efficiently in a warm, rather than a cold, environment. Warming up increases the temperature of the muscle so that energy production is more efficient, and prepares the body for action with an increase in heart rate, oxygen uptake and blood flow to the muscles.

Warming down is all about bringing the body back to its resting state steadily, giving time for any lactic acid to be removed from the muscles, and also offering a few important moments of psychological reflection on the run that has just occurred.

WARMING UP

While warming up is essential for sprinters involved in high-intensity anaerobic activities, it could be argued that it has a lesser role in endurance activities such as marathon training. However, training runs put an immediate stress on the body, particularly if the session is at a high intensity. In my experience, runners often start a training run following a period of inactivity – after a night of sleeping for example, during a lunch break or after a day spent sitting in an office, or after a long commute home. Sudden exercise without preparation can be a cardiovascular and muscular shock that at best results in poor performance, and at worst injury. I generally find that there are two different approaches to a training-run warm up. The first is to have a dedicated pre-run period for warming up, which should involve some light jogging for 5–10 minutes to raise body temperature,

followed by some gentle stretching of the leg muscles, particularly the calves. Muscles are more supple and easy to stretch when warm, so it is best to delay stretching until after the jogging has increased muscle temperature. The second option is to incorporate your warm-up into the first part of your training run – this means setting off at a slow pace to give your body the chance to ease into the activity, and being prepared to stop after a few minutes to do some stretching. This

> **'Warming up increases the temperature of the muscle so that energy production is more efficient, and prepares the body for action with an increase in heart rate, oxygen uptake and blood flow to the muscles.'**

can be either dynamic – incorporating rapid movements – or static, where the muscle is gently stretched with minimal movement. Although research is not clear which is best, the lower intensities of marathon training and racing when compared with other more dynamic sports, suggests that static stretching is a safer and lower risk option for most marathon runners. As your training for a marathon makes progress, and race day gets ever closer, the impact of an injury becomes greater, so while warming up can at times seem like an unnecessary distraction from the run ahead, if it prevents an injury it can make all the difference between a marathon completion and non-completion.

WARMING DOWN

At the end of a training run, particularly one that has been at a moderate or high intensity, your body's metabolic rate will have increased, and there will almost certainly be some lactic acid in the muscles and blood. While there is always a temptation to stop

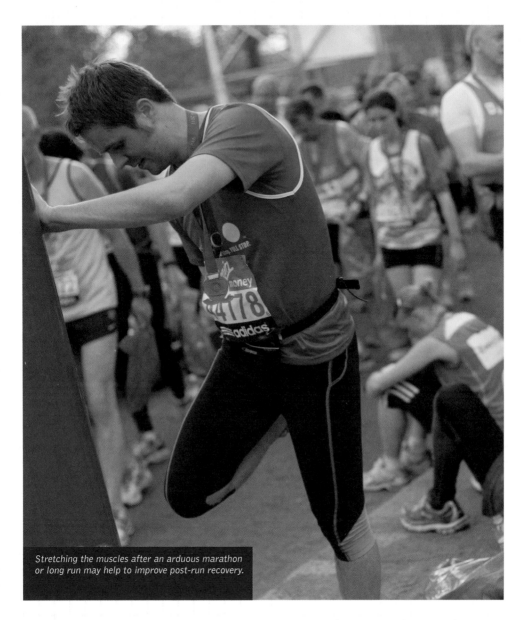

Stretching the muscles after an arduous marathon or long run may help to improve post-run recovery.

completely once the run is over, spending a few minutes slowly jogging while the body's systems return to normal can help to clear any lactic acid from the blood and may reduce stiffness or soreness the following day. Since the muscles will be warm and supple, this can be a good time to do some stretching to improve flexibility.

Warming up and warming down should be seen as an integral part of a training plan, not an optional extra. Together, they contribute to injury prevention, enhanced training performance, and improved recovery. The time invested in doing both can make the marginal difference between sustained high-quality training, and an injury that threatens training and race day.

'Warming down is all about bringing the body back to its resting state steadily, giving time for any lactic acid to be removed from the muscles, and also offering a few important moments of psychological reflection.'

RUNNING IN DIFFERENT WEATHER CONDITIONS

Running in a range of weather conditions provides different challenges and experiences. Coping with, and using these conditions to enhance training and racing is a factor in achieving marathon success.

Most major marathon races are held in the spring or autumn, when the more extreme conditions of summer and winter are avoided. However, this means that the majority of marathon training takes place in more challenging conditions, and, in Section One we explored the science-based differences of hot- and cold-weather running. Now we will consider how best to cope with running in, and preparing for, different climatic conditions.

Spring marathons can cause problems, since the warm (or even hot) conditions that could be encountered are often a physiological and psychological shock after training through the colder winter months. I have run London Marathons in April where race day has been one of the warmest of the year, and far hotter than any encountered previously during my preparations, leaving many runners unprepared and often unable to cope with the unexpected heat.

Your marathon training needs to prepare you for this possibility, so it is important to use every opportunity to adapt to warmer conditions – a process scientists call 'acclimation'. Check the weather forecast, and make sure you train on days that are warm during the weeks before the race – this helps with acclimation, and prepares you for the feeling of warm running. Wearing extra layers helps to create a personal 'microclimate' of warmth, even on colder days, which tricks the body into acclimation. Hats and wet tops can help, since they restrict heat loss into the external environment. I like to think of these sessions as acclimation runs. Even if race day turns out to be cooler than

expected, they are still a great investment and worth doing at least once a week during the final four to five weeks of marathon training, since scientists have shown that training in warm conditions can be just as beneficial as altitude training. A sensible approach is needed though, and if an acclimation strategy that involves wearing extra layers builds up too much heat, be prepared to slow down or remove layers to avoid becoming too hot.

Running in cold conditions presents less of a challenge, although initially

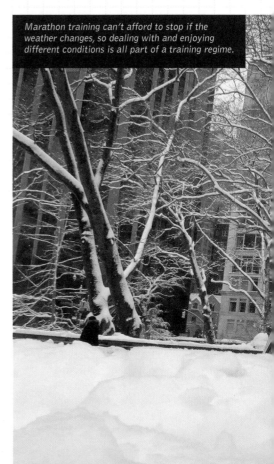

Marathon training can't afford to stop if the weather changes, so dealing with and enjoying different conditions is all part of a training regime.

peripheral parts of the body such as the arms and legs will feel cold. However, the energy produced from running will soon generate heat even on the coldest days, so it is important not to start wearing too many layers, otherwise you will quickly feel hot and uncomfortable (unless, of course, you are doing an acclimation run). On really cold days, running in a hat or gloves retains body heat, but I find that these are never really necessary after a couple of miles, at which point body temperature and blood flow will have increased. In extreme conditions, when there is snow or ice on the ground, safety and injury avoidance are the main priority, and this may even be time to venture into a local gym to find a treadmill.

Wet-weather running tends to be more of a psychological challenge than a physical one. It's hard to be enthusiastic about heading out of the door when the rain is falling and the pavements are wet. The first few steps are always the hardest – once you are wet and have generated body heat, things improve. Be careful not to wear clothing that will easily absorb moisture, since this will become heavy and uncomfortable and could cause chafing. If possible, avoid puddles that will get your feet wet, since this can easily cause sores and blisters.

Training for autumn marathons during the summer months offers longer daylight hours and the chance to plan training around the weather. On really hot days, avoid long runs and over-exertion – shorter, interval sessions may be better, confining longer runs to the cooler early morning or evenings. As already mentioned, get into the habit of weighing yourself before and after a training session, and replacing each 1kg (2.2lb) lost with 1 litre (1¾ pints) of fluid.

Running in different weather conditions adds variety, and can completely change the experience of doing the same route. Taking sensible precautions and adapting your training to the conditions means that variable weather should enhance, not hinder, your marathon training and racing.

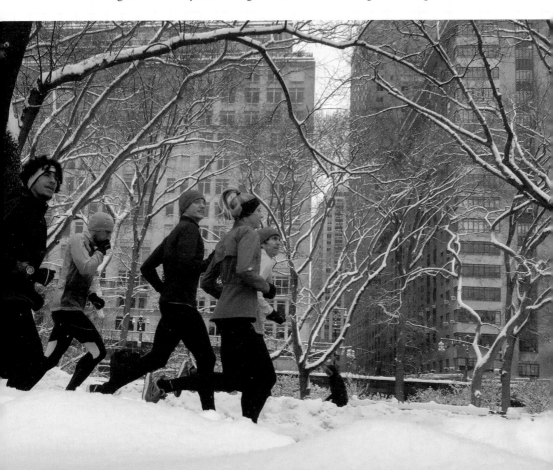

CROSS-TRAINING

Marathons involve running, but there are times when alternative activities, or cross-training, have a role to play. Knowing when and how to use cross-training is important for all marathon runners.

At some point during your marathon training, something will almost certainly go wrong that will disrupt your plans, the most common being illness or injury. The first thing to remember is not to panic – there are steps that can be taken to reduce the damage, and still ensure that you can successfully run 26.2 miles.

In Section One on page 58, the importance of specificity in a marathon-training programme was highlighted, and of course this means that running has to be prioritised. But if injury strikes, and running is no longer possible, all is not lost. I like to consider marathon training as the development of two distinct areas of the body. The first is the 'central' cardiovascular system – the lungs, heart and oxygen-transport system. The second is the 'peripheral' muscles, tendons and ligaments that are involved in the physical process

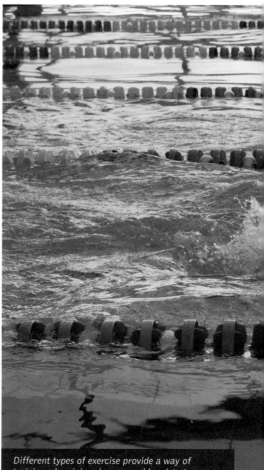

Different types of exercise provide a way of training when injured, or can add variety to a training programme.

'Using cross-training as a 'running substitute' should ideally only be seen as a short-term measure that allows an injury the chance to heal and, if the injury permits it, it is a better alternative to complete rest.'

of running and energy production. While running develops both, it is the peripheral area that will only respond effectively to the specific demands of running – other forms of activity will provide a challenge to the cardiovascular system, though they will not have the same specific impact on the anatomical parts of the body used when running.

Cross-training could include a range of activities, but of course if you are injured,

there may only be certain exercises that are manageable. Cycling and swimming both eliminate many of the stresses and impact forces that result from running, and even though they will not overload the running-specific peripheral parts of the body, they will help to maintain central, cardiovascular fitness. Using cross-training as a 'running substitute' should ideally only be seen as a short-term measure that allows an injury the chance to heal and, if the injury permits it, it is a better alternative to complete rest, and should allow for a more effective resumption of training once the recovery process is complete.

It is possible to incorporate cross-training into a marathon programme, this can help add variety and an opportunity

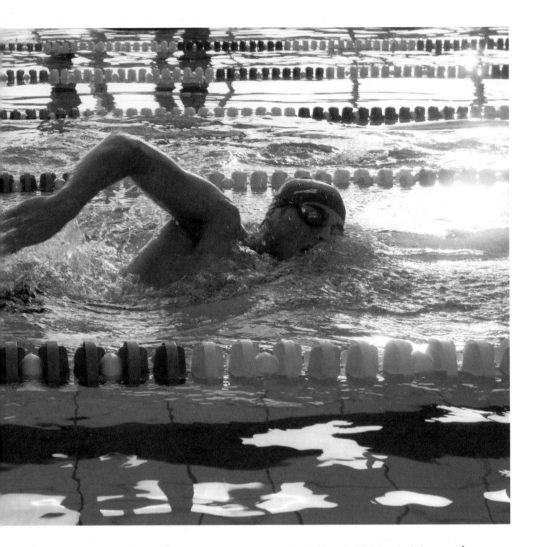

for recovery, or can be used as a more regular training component to develop core strength and stability. When used for general conditioning, cross-training can help improve strength and reduce the risk of injury, although if time is short – which probably it is for most non-elite runners – running needs to remain the central component of marathon training. It is also important to select the type of cross-training carefully. As your marathon training progresses and your body adapts, you will become conditioned to running repetitively in a straight line. Adding variety with a different activity, such as squash, tennis or even soccer, which involves twisting, turning and short bursts of high-intensity

activity is an invitation to injury, and over the years I have heard far too many stories of weeks of training being undone by the mistaken participation in an activity or sport that the runner's body was unable to cope with. Running has to remain the focal point of a marathon training programme. Cross-training can add some variety to training, but care should be taken to ensure that it does not involve activities that are going to provide unnecessary or unusual stresses on the body. Cross-training does have a role for an injured runner: to improve general strength and conditioning, and for injury prevention. It can also help reduce the decline in fitness – particularly within the cardiovascular system that occurs when injury strikes.

Injuries are a constant threat, but can be prevented with planning and a sensible approach to training.

INJURY PREVENTION AND LISTENING TO YOUR BODY

Injury is one of the biggest threats to a marathon-training programme. But there are steps that can be taken to reduce injury risk and ensure that training continues unhindered.

For marathon runners of all abilities, injuries are an occupational hazard. The relentless impact from many miles of training will occasionally take its toll, and result in a breakdown of tissue or bone that will inevitably cause some disruption to training, and may even pose a threat to race day itself.

As is the case for most medical conditions, prevention is better – and easier – than cure, and there are plenty of simple steps that runners can take to reduce the risk of an injury occurring.

PREHAB

It is becoming increasingly common for runners to seek specialist medical help from an expert such as a chartered physiotherapist who can conduct a series of simple screening tests at the outset of a

MYTH: *MARATHON RUNNING IS BAD FOR YOU*

Watch any marathon, and you will almost certainly see runners hobbling, grimacing and even bleeding as they struggle to reach the finish line. 'Marathons must be bad for you' is a phrase frequently uttered by observers with great authority, but these are often individuals sitting in front of a TV, whose main form of exertion is to pick up the remote control.

Of course marathon running is tough, but any pain and discomfort associated with completing the distance is normally temporary, disappearing long before the euphoria that comes from going the distance. Just occasionally, there are more tragic consequences, with runners dying as a result of their exertions. Sadly, this is inevitable and in some ways not a surprise when mass events attract many thousands of individuals all exerting themselves for many hours. There are often underlying reasons for marathon fatalities, which have been triggered by running, rather than caused by it. For the vast majority of individuals, the health benefits gained as a consequence of training for, and running, a marathon, far outweigh the risks, and every year many thousands of people will lead healthier, and possibly longer, lives as a result of marathons.

That said, running many miles definitely places stresses on the body, particularly the lower legs and knees, and this is why sensible rather than obsessive training is important, combined with appropriate footwear and nutrition to reduce the risk of injury and long-term wear and tear. On the flip side, marathon training contributes to muscle strength, bone health and cardiovascular fitness in a far better way than any medication, and while there will always be exceptions, for the vast majority, marathons benefit rather than harm the human body.

training programme. As opposed to the more common term of 'rehab' used for post-injury recovery, this 'prehab' identifies any weaknesses or imbalances that may increase the risk of an injury occurring, and should include remedial exercises to reduce your injury risk.

FOOTWEAR

It may seem obvious, but wearing proper running shoes that are comfortable, provide cushioning and support, and that suit your running style, is crucial. Visit a specialist running shop and seek expert advice on what type of shoe best meets your needs.

MILEAGE

Trying to do too much, too soon, is probably one of the most common causes of injury with marathon runners.

The injury risk is high at the start of a programme, when enthusiasm combines with a lack of running background and conditioning to place demands on the muscles, tendons, bones and ligaments that they are not used to, and this can quickly lead to breakdown and injury. But it can also occur during a programme, if runners progress the volume and intensity of their training at too rapid a rate. Training will cause minor damage to tissues, and it is only after they repair and regenerate that they become stronger. Failing to allow sufficient time for this to happen just results in a gradual breakdown rather than continuous improvement, and injury quickly follows.

NUTRITION

Keeping your body properly fuelled through a diet that is high in carbohydrate, with plenty of fresh fruit, vegetables and variety will fight tiredness and maintain your immune system. Having enough energy to run properly makes you less likely to incur an injury than when running on empty, which causes consequent fatigue and loss of coordination.

SLEEP

It is during our sleeping hours that the body repairs and responds to the rigours of training. Get into the habit of sleeping well, even if it means going to bed earlier than you may be used to – this means efficient time management since adding 'running time' into your life will inevitably put more pressure on your day. Avoid the temptation to miss out on sleep in an attempt to squeeze everything in.

LISTEN TO YOUR BODY

As your marathon training progresses, you will inevitably feel soreness and aching. This is normal, and is a sign that your body is changing and adapting to long-distance running. But there will be times when these aches seem worse than normal, or are focussed on a specific part of your anatomy, such as your calf muscle or Achilles tendon. This is invariably a warning signal that you cannot and should not overlook. Missing a few days' training while an injury is minor is much better than training through the pain, making the injury chronic and being faced with having to miss weeks of training rather than days. If you are injured, seek early advice from an expert such as your doctor or a chartered physiotherapist and be prepared to rest and avoid making the injury worse.

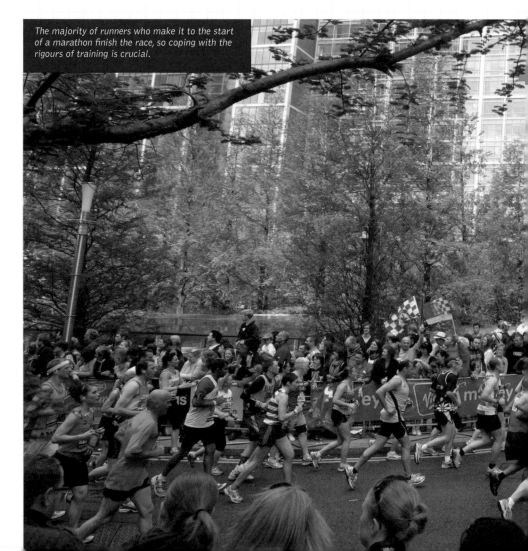

The majority of runners who make it to the start of a marathon finish the race, so coping with the rigours of training is crucial.

MYTH: *HEART RATE MONITORS ARE ESSENTIAL*

Thirty years ago, the only way to measure heart rate accurately while running was in a laboratory, with wires attached to various parts of the body, linked to a large heart rate monitor. The practicalities made measuring and monitoring heart rate anywhere else cumbersome and impossible.

Over the years, technology has advanced, initially enabling runners to monitor their heart rate from devices resembling a very large watch, to much smaller units that not only provide real-time feedback, but also enable data to be stored and retrospectively analysed. As a consequence, it has become common for scientists and coaching manuals to recommend heart rate training zones for marathon running and racing, which have

been adopted by many seeking to base their training on science rather than subjectivity.

However, heart rate data can be notoriously fickle, changing with age, climate and from one person to another. Sticking obsessively to a particular heart rate zone can work well, or it can cause chaos, and for most runners, the best advice is to use heart rate data merely as a guide. It helps to give a feel for training intensity, but should not dictate it, and it is important to remember that many hundreds of thousands of people have successfully trained for and run marathons without the use of heart rate technology. They are an optional extra, rather than essential part of the marathon runner's kit bag.

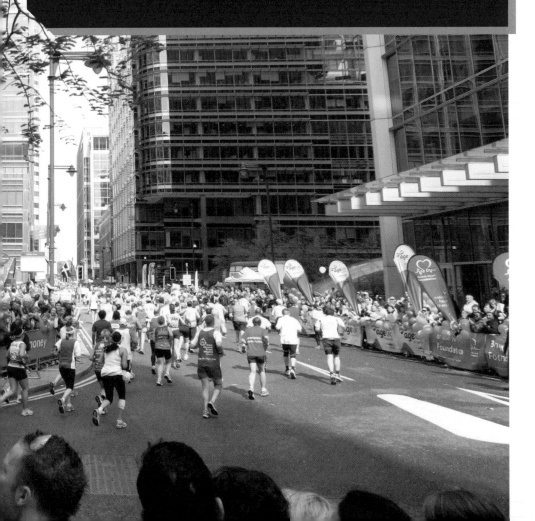

GOAL SETTING

How fast can you go? It's a question asked by all marathon runners, but how do you make sure your race-day goal is realistic and achievable?

As race day approaches, it is time to start setting a goal for your forthcoming marathon. This must be realistic and based on performances during your marathon preparation. Of course, the main goal for any marathon runner should be to complete the 26.2-mile distance, but over the years, I have spoken to many hundreds of runners during the last few days before a marathon, and almost all have had a target time in mind. Surprisingly, though, far fewer have had a strategy in place to achieve their time, or even understood what their running pace needs to be in order to achieve it. This simply doesn't work: once you have determined a realistic target time, it is vital that you understand how this translates into running speed.

As your training progresses, your body will adapt and improve, and it is important that your race-day goal reflects this physiological transition into a marathon runner. At the same time, setting a goal that is achievable is crucial, and to do this you must have an understanding of the distances and pace that you are covering in training.

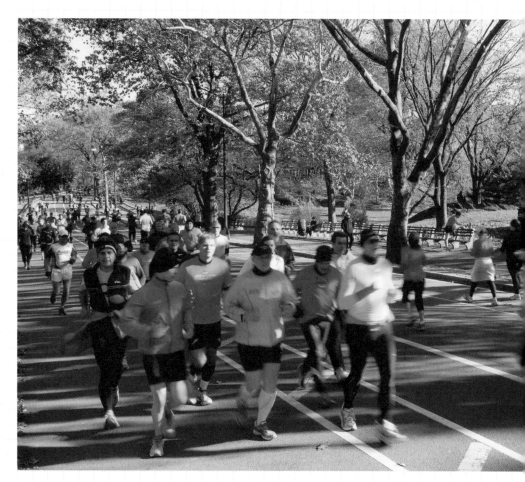

Working out your training pace is quite straightforward – simply divide the time your run has taken by the distance covered. But it is only when your training extends to longer distances towards the end of a plan that your training pace can be used to realistically predict a marathon time. As an example, if you can sustain 8 minutes per mile for a 10-mile run, but are tired at the end, it is highly unlikely that this pace – or even faster – will be possible over 26.2 miles. However, if the same speed is manageable over 20 miles in training, it is more likely that a pace that is not much slower will be feasible for a marathon.

To gain a better understanding of how your training is progressing, and to provide a more valuable indicator of race-day performance, I always advise runners to include at least two organised distance

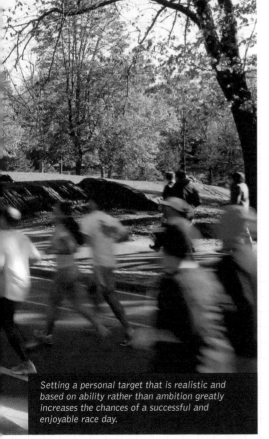

Setting a personal target that is realistic and based on ability rather than ambition greatly increases the chances of a successful and enjoyable race day.

'An often-used general guideline is to take a half-marathon time, double it, then add 15-20 minutes to predict marathon time, allowing for a drop in pace of just under 1 minute per mile for the longer distance.'

races as part of their marathon training. When mass-participation events are on the horizon, many race organisers will capitalise by arranging events during the weeks before a marathon over shorter distances – the most common being half-marathons and 20-mile races. Entering pre-marathon races has a number of advantages. Firstly, it gets runners used to running with others and to the whole experience of race day, which can be daunting for first-timers. Secondly, they are a great way of completing a long training run in company, often with the support of drinks stations, which further helps race-day preparations. Finally, they provide a useful predictor of your race-day goal and what 26.2-mile time you could achieve. An often-used general guideline is to take a half-marathon time, double it, then add 15–20 minutes to predict marathon time, allowing for a drop in pace of just under 1 minute per mile for the longer distance.

In 1997, a research engineer, Pete Riegel, applied a mathematical formula to marathon-time prediction, which can be used to give an indication of race-day target time:

Marathon time = $TD \times (26.2/D)^{1.06}$

Where D is the distance of the training run/race
And TD is the time (minutes) of the training run/race

Of course this does not take into account training status, experience or all-important pacing, all of which will impact on final finishing time. However, it does provide a guide around which a realistic goal can be set for race day, which can then be used to calculate a sensible pacing strategy. Race-day goal setting, and pace setting to achieve that goal, are essential parts of race-day preparation, and unless done properly, jeopardise many weeks and months of training.

COPING WITH ILLNESS

Everyone gets ill at some point, and dealing with illness while training is common. Learning how to cope so that it is manageable and not critical, is very important for all marathon runners.

In the same way that injuries are an occupational hazard for marathon runners, so too is illness. After all, not many of us go through a six-month period without some form of illness, no matter how minor, so the chances of staying completely healthy and illness-free while training for a marathon are slim. In fact, there is even evidence to suggest that the risk of some illnesses is actually greater among marathon runners, since the strenuous exercise associated with the many miles of training can have an impact on the body's immune system, making it less able to fight off infection, particularly after long training runs or intensive periods of training.

As with an injury, it is important to listen to your body, and if you feel unwell or think an illness is on the near-horizon, don't resist taking some time off from your training. I have seen runners determined to train through an illness, and in doing so simply make matters far worse. A few days off to recover can give the body's immune system time to fight back, and may well prevent a more serious illness occurring.

Understanding when an illness means calling a temporary halt to training helps to ensure that you don't exacerbate the situation. At the first sign of a raised temperature, sickness or stomach problems, take time off. An elevated temperature is a clear signal that all is not well – perhaps as a result of an infection or virus – and continuing to train is more likely to do harm than good.

Colds and lung problems are also common, especially if training occurs during

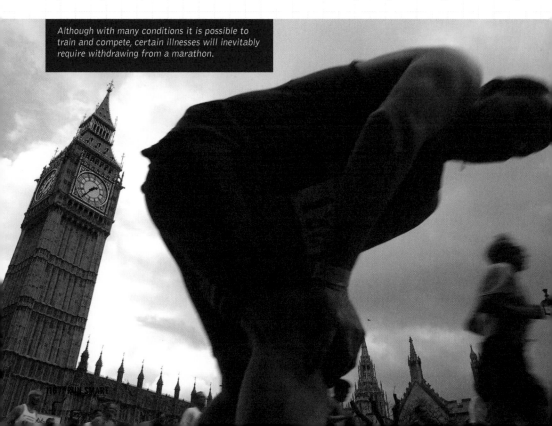

Although with many conditions it is possible to train and compete, certain illnesses will inevitably require withdrawing from a marathon.

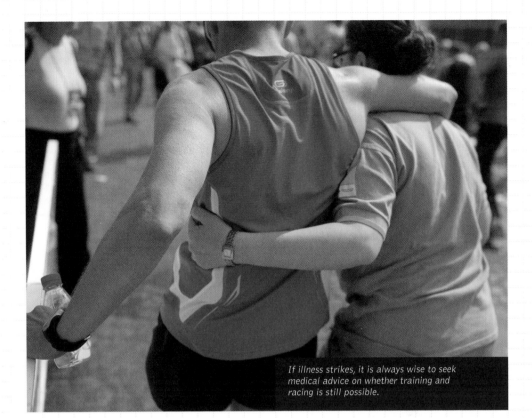

If illness strikes, it is always wise to seek medical advice on whether training and racing is still possible.

the winter months. A possible reason for their frequency is explained by the results from studies of marathon runners that have shown that after long runs the risk of upper respiratory tract infections is increased, almost certainly because the immune system remains temporarily supressed for up to 24 hours. The general guideline for this sort of illness is that if the cold remains confined to the head – a blocked nose and sinuses – then it is fine to continue training. However, if it extends to the lungs, with coughing and mucous, it is time to stop and rest. Remember that running results in significant volumes of air entering and leaving the lungs each minute, increasing the capacity to bring even more bacteria or viruses into the body. Giving your lungs a chance to recuperate is the best option, but if symptoms persist for more than a week to 10 days, it will be worth visiting your doctor for medical advice.

As with an injury, if illness occurs mid-programme it should not be too problematic, and simply result in a minor disruption of your training plans. However, when either occurs during the critical last few weeks – or even days – before a marathon, the situation is far more serious. Anyone with a condition that is likely to be made worse by running a marathon should seriously consider withdrawal, and many major races will allow an entry to be deferred until the following year, even up to 24 hours before race day. However, if the injury or illness has been short term, and had a disruptive rather than debilitating impact on training, then there is still the option to complete the race, provided you are confident that you are fit and well enough to do so. It will mean revising your goals – downwards of course – and accepting that the finish time that you may have aspired to before the problem is no longer possible. But if your aim is to complete the distance, and possibly achieve a lifetime goal or raise money for charity by doing so, then all may not be lost if a sensible and slower strategy is adopted for race day.

OVERTRAINING

Marathon training treads a fine line between overload and overtraining. Prevention and reaction are key if overtraining is to be avoided or overcome.

It is easy to confuse overtraining with tiredness. However, there are very few marathon runners who don't become tired as a result of their training, whereas overtraining occurs when the body fails to recover properly from the rigours of that training, and can occur in up to 10 per cent of runners who are preparing hard for an event such as a marathon, unless steps are taken to prevent it. One of the possible causes of overtraining is the natural endorphins produced by running, which can have the same effect as any drug, and become addictive. The body craves exercise, and in the case of marathon training, a feeling of 'more is better' takes over. When this is accompanied by limited recovery time, the symptoms of overtraining soon follow.

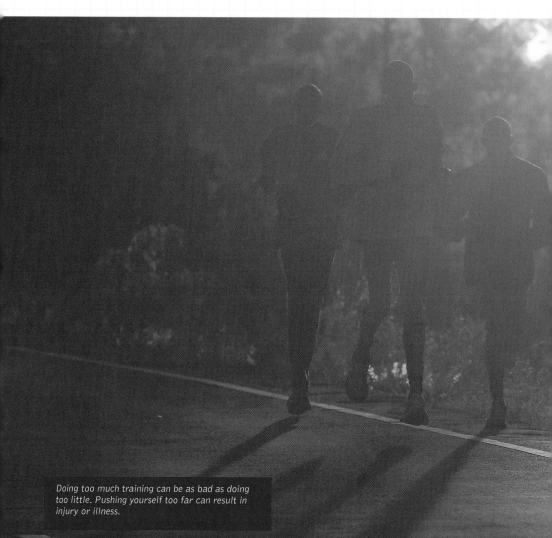

Doing too much training can be as bad as doing too little. Pushing yourself too far can result in injury or illness.

'Overtraining is often accompanied by feelings of fatigue even when not running, sometimes apparent at the start of the day. Other symptoms are a loss of appetite, an increased incidence of injuries, poor sleep patterns, lethargy and a loss of enthusiasm for running.'

As we have seen, overload is essential if the body is going to adapt and improve, but much of this adaptation occurs during the recovery time within a training programme. If the balance is wrong, and too much overload combines with too little recovery, training becomes harder. Instead of experiencing gradual improvements, runners see a steady and inexplicable decline in their performances, and fail to recover fully between sessions.

As with illness and injury, there are warning signs that should be recognised. The most obvious is a drop in performance, which many runners will try to redress by training even harder and cutting down still further on recovery, something that only serves to make matters worse. Overtraining is often accompanied by feelings of fatigue even when not running, sometimes apparent at the start of the day. Other symptoms are a loss of appetite, an increased incidence of injuries, poor sleep patterns, lethargy and a loss of

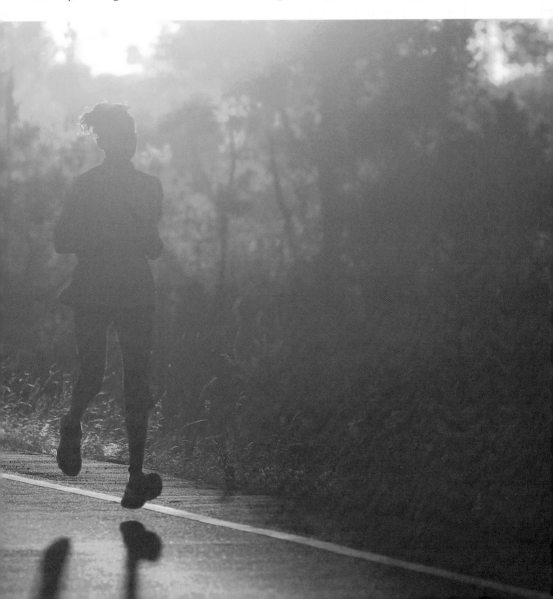

Running at the right pace and frequency for you, and no one else, is essential if overtraining is to be avoided.

enthusiasm for running. Mood changes are common, with periods of irritability and even mild depression, and there may also be muscle pains that take a long time to resolve, and a higher-than-normal incidence of minor illnesses such as colds and infections.

Prevention is of course better than cure, and this is why a good training programme will prescribe both high- and low-intensity sessions, interspersed with sensible periods of recovery. Any desire to do more than the programme suggests, or your body feels capable of coping with, should be resisted. It is also important to maintain a healthy diet, with plenty of carbohydrate and nutrients to support the recovery process and your immune system.

One simple way of monitoring for overtraining is to check your resting heart rate at the start of each day. This is best done while still in bed, and the value should be written down and monitored over time. Don't be concerned about a variation between one day and the next, but if there is a consistent increase over a period of four or five days, then it suggests that you may not be recovering properly, and need to take action.

'It is important to note that running that causes overtraining in one person could have no impact on another – differences in age, sex and fitness levels all impact on susceptibility – so don't compare yourself with other people.'

The simplest and most effective thing to do is to reduce your training load and increase your recovery time – this may also be a good time to introduce some cross-training to give your body a further chance to recover. It is important to recognise that you don't need to stop training completely, and so long as there is sufficient rest and recovery time, after a week or so most marathon runners should be capable of resuming their normal training, provided that the same mistakes are avoided.

It is also important to note that running that causes overtraining in one person could have no impact on another – differences in age, sex and fitness levels all impact on susceptibility – so don't compare yourself with other people. The most important thing is to prevent it happening by listening to your own body, and to react quickly if symptoms develop.

MYTH: *YOU SHOULD NOT RUN MORE THAN TWO OR THREE MARATHONS A YEAR*

The arduous nature of marathon training and racing results in many positive adaptations to the human body, together with the development of mental resilience that is vital for the times when things get tough. Because of this, most runners rightly feel the need to take time off after a marathon to give themselves the chance to recover. As a consequence, there is a view that at most two or three marathons per year are feasible, while for many they are an annual – or once-a-lifetime – challenge.

However, the many miles of marathon training, and the completion of the distance, mean that once a week or so has passed, most runners, especially first-timers, are fitter than they have ever been, and have certainly achieved 'marathon fitness'. This

post-race period offers an opportunity to preserve that fitness and put it to use again in the not-too-distant future, and within weeks, rather than months, another marathon could be possible. Indeed, as individuals seek to push back the boundaries of human endurance still further, there are those who complete numerous marathons on consecutive days.

Elite runners looking to push their bodies to the limit may well only be capable of producing their peak marathon performance on two or at most three occasions a year, and the same is true of those who consistently race marathons for personal-best times. However, for runners wanting to complete the distance, more regular, if not fast, marathon running is certainly possible.

MYTH: *LACTIC ACID CAUSES POST-RACE SORENESS*

For a number of days after completing a marathon, runners are likely to experience some degree of muscle soreness. For some this is nothing more than minor discomfort, for others it can be quite debilitating. This soreness is a by-product of fatigue, and the exertion associated with a marathon. However, the cause of this fatigue is, in the majority of cases, a result of a loss of fluid and/or energy (glycogen). Unlike runners racing distances at a higher intensity, it is unlikely to be caused by a build-up of lactic acid, which is a by-product of energy production when the intensity of exercise is high.

Scientists have found that the great majority of marathon runners complete the distance at a pace that enables energy in the muscles to be produced in the presence of

oxygen – or aerobically – and as a result only small amounts of lactic acid are produced. Elite marathon runners are able to run the distance at a higher intensity, but even this is unlikely to produce the levels of lactic acid seen after races over shorter distances.

The temporary muscle soreness experienced after running a marathon is due to minor damage to the muscle fibres, and inflammation within the muscle, and not as a result of lactic acid. The muscles consist of many millions of tiny myofilaments, and these link together like cogs, which work together to control muscle movement. Each stride action puts these myofilaments under stress, and can even pull them apart, and it is this that eventually results in pain and muscle soreness.

THE FINAL WEEKS AND TAPERING

The final weeks and days before a marathon are critical – get it wrong, and all the hard training will be wasted. But get it right, and you will start the race fully prepared for the 26.2 miles ahead.

Running a marathon is not like revising for an exam – you cannot cram everything in at the last minute. In fact, the opposite is the case, since the final two to three weeks leading up to race day should be a time when the intensity and volume of training is reduced, and you prepare yourself mentally and physically for the challenge ahead.

The final long run should be no closer than two weeks before race day, but this is not necessarily your longest run. I normally suggest that the longest training run – taking you to at least 20 miles, and ideally a little way beyond – should be three weeks before the race for first-timers, but could be a fortnight before for those with more experience. Three weeks builds in a safety margin for recovery

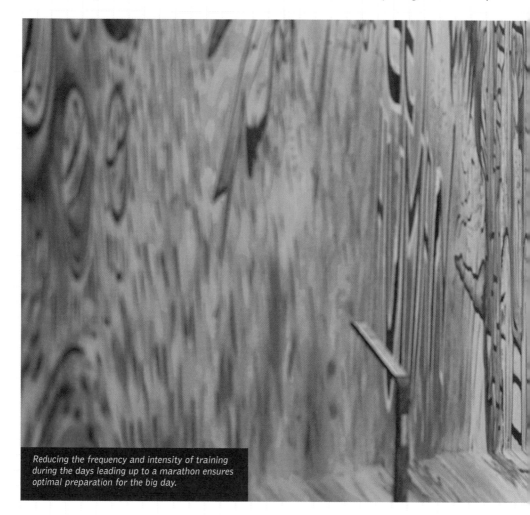

Reducing the frequency and intensity of training during the days leading up to a marathon ensures optimal preparation for the big day.

in case of minor injuries or muscle soreness, while two weeks works well as a pre-race confidence boost, but does provide limited recovery time.

The worst mistake a runner can make is to continue with a high-mileage strategy in the final two weeks before the race. This risks injury and fatigue, and seldom works as a substitute for proper training over the preceding weeks and months. If your longest run is three weeks before race day, it can be followed by a further long run of 16–18 miles with two weeks to go, then a slow, easy run of around 10 miles with one week remaining. This is a good time to get a feel for your marathon pace, and use these final runs to think through your approach to race day and, most importantly, visualise yourself crossing the finish line. If you haven't done so already, practise drinking and taking gels while running, making sure that if there are branded sports drinks or gels on course, you have tried them and are comfortable with their taste. It is also a good time to run in your race-day apparel so that you are certain that everything fits and there are no expected seams that could cause chafing.

It is not a good idea to stop running completely during the final days of

'If you haven't done so already, practise drinking and taking gels while running, making sure that if there are branded sports drinks or gels on course, you have tried them and are comfortable with their taste.'

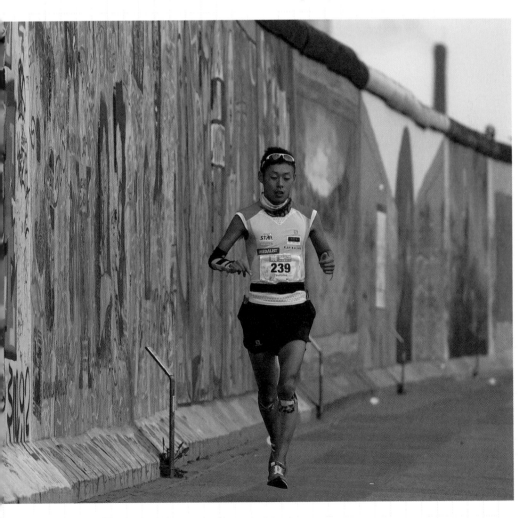

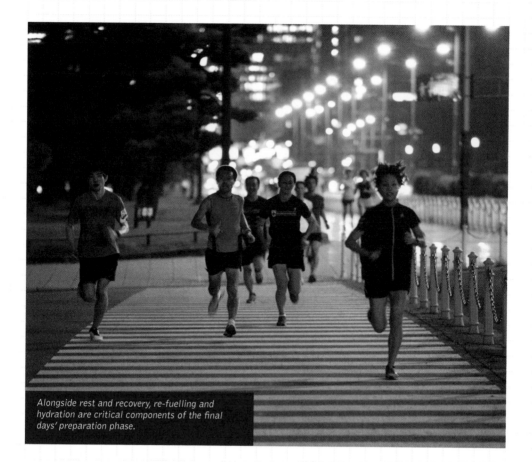

Alongside rest and recovery, re-fuelling and hydration are critical components of the final days' preparation phase.

preparation, but the distance should be no more than 3–5 miles, at a slow pace. Be prepared for a shock – your legs may feel tired and heavy – almost certainly as a result of glycogen stores building up in your muscles, which is a good sign, and nothing to be concerned about. Make sure you run on flat ground, limiting the chance of twisting an ankle, and keep your speed low so that fat, rather than glycogen makes the main contribution to energy production.

This is the time to focus on your race-day fuelling strategy, with carbohydrate forming the main part of your diet. It is important to stay properly hydrated, so keep checking your urine to ensure that it is a pale, straw colour. I usually advise runners to keep carbohydrate snacks with them during the final two or three days before the race – foods such as jelly babies and bananas work well – and use them to keep energy stores topped up. The combination of a decrease in training load and a high-carbohydrate diet will ensure that your glycogen stores are not only fully charged, but 'super-compensated'. This is the term used when glycogen levels are elevated to above-normal levels – something that used to be achieved from 'carbohydrate loading', but which we now know occurs when training is reduced while a high-carbohydrate diet is eaten.

The final weeks and days are a time for fine-tuning, ensuring that you stand on the start line ready and able to capitalise on the hard work that has gone into many weeks and months of preparation. Rest rather than running is the priority as the 26.2-mile challenge looms large.

'The combination of a decrease in training load and a high-carbohydrate diet will ensure that your glycogen stores are not only fully charged, but 'super-compensated.'

MYTH: **ALCOHOL IS BANNED**

The side effects from alcohol consumption are not conducive to running. Dehydration, impaired decision making and a build-up of toxins in the blood all make running after drinking alcohol difficult at best, and at worst, not possible at all. Furthermore, alcohol contains calories that are of little use as an energy source for runners. Each gram of alcohol contains 7 calories of energy, and a bottle of wine with an alcohol content of 13 per cent will contain almost 700 calories from alcohol alone, so excessive consumption can quickly result in weight gain.

Many runners decide to omit alcohol from their diet during training, and this is undoubtedly beneficial. But is it essential? The answer is 'no', provided that alcohol consumption is in moderation, and not at a level that has a negative impact on training or recovery. The very nature of marathon training means that energy expenditure will rise, and this can counter the extra calories consumed from alcohol. Marathon training is also tough both mentally and physically, so taking time to relax and wind down with the odd glass of wine or beer is perfectly acceptable.

Consuming alcohol in the days before the marathon itself is somewhat different, and should be done with great caution. Many runners will abstain from alcohol as race day approaches, and certainly on the night before. Ensuring that the body tapers properly and is fully prepared for race day is critical; everything possible should be done to arrive at the start line in the best possible condition, optimising all of the hard work and effort that has gone into marathon training.

MYTH: **EAT AS MANY CARBS AS POSSIBLE BEFORE RACE DAY**

There is no doubt that carbs are crucial for marathon success. Stored as glycogen, they provide the essential fuel needed to complete the distance, and under normal circumstances, runners will have enough glycogen in their muscles and liver to provide around 1800–2000 calories of energy. However, most runners need 3000 calories of energy to run 26.2 miles, so as a result there is an energy deficit that can be met by eating extra carbohydrate before race day.

But how much extra is needed, and can you eat too much? With normal energy reserves of around 1800 calories, and an energy demand of 3000 calories, the additional energy that the body needs is around 1200 calories. However, with sensible pacing, a proportion of this can come from the body's much larger energy reserves of body fat. Assuming this is around 20 per cent of the total requirement, or 600 calories, the deficit is reduced to just 400 calories. Each gram of carbohydrate provides 4 calories of energy, so the extra carbohydrate requirement is not much more than 100 grams. As an example, this equates to four medium-sized bananas or 400g (14oz) of cooked pasta.

In conclusion, while of course eating carbohydrate before a marathon is necessary as glycogen stores must be as full as possible, closer examination of the energy demands of marathon running, and the important role that fat reserves play when the race is paced properly, show that even when it comes to the all-important carbs, you can have too much of a good thing!

Marathon training is tough, but running with the support of others can make training easy and help with motivation.

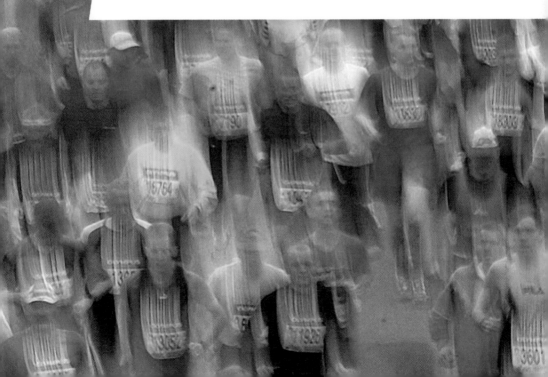

SECTION THREE
RACE PREPARATION AND RACE DAY

The day of the race is nearly here and your mood is likely to be a mixture of nerves and excitement. This section will show you how to manage such critical areas as nutrition, hydration and pacing. It will also explain how best to deal with a crisis if things do go wrong.

PRE-RACE PLANNING

With race day looming, proper planning is essential if things are going to go well. Overlook one critical planning element, and all of your hard work could be jeopardised.

I once worked with an international coach who was a great advocate of the 'five ps' – 'poor preparation produces poor performance' – and as a consequence his planning during the build-up to an important competition was impeccable. Marathons are no exception, and planning your last few days and hours is critical if race day is going to be successful. Here are a few of the things you should think about and plan before the race:

HOW DO I GET MY NUMBER?

Will it be sent in the post, or do I need to collect it? If it is being collected, where do I need to be and by when? Most major marathons have a pre-race expo where runners collect their numbers, and you should decide when to attend, and how to get there. If possible, I always advise runners not to go on the day before the race, since it is all too easy to become tired and dehydrated from walking around an indoor exhibition arena.

Get race day right and your marathon will be a great experience. But get it wrong, and it could be a day you will want to forget!

WHEN AND WHERE DOES THE RACE START?

I have come across runners who, with less than 24 hours to go, have no idea where or when their marathon starts. Of course this is more of an issue with major races in cities that people are not familiar with, but it is essential that you know where to be and when to be there weeks, rather than days, in advance.

HOW WILL I GET TO THE START AND WHEN SHOULD I BE THERE?

Plan your route to the start carefully, and seek advice on the best mode of transport. For big races, roads are often closed near the start, but if you intend to travel by train, check train times and even whether your train line is running – marathons are often on Sundays when some lines are

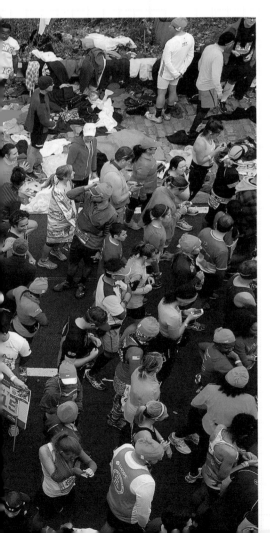

closed. I normally recommend that runners get to the start at least one-and-a-half hours before the gun goes, giving a bit of spare time in case things go wrong, as well as time to sort out clothing and to queue for the toilet!

HOW WILL I COLLECT MY CLOTHING AT THE FINISH?

Some marathons start and finish in the same place whereas others finish some distance from the start. If necessary, race organisers will arrange baggage transfer from the start to the finish, but you must check in advance how this works, and possible restrictions on the size and type of bag that will be carried.

WHERE WILL I MEET FAMILY AND FRIENDS AFTERWARDS?

Many races have repatriation areas where you can meet friends and family afterwards, but if this is not the case you should find a prearranged meeting point. While it is tempting to use mobile phones, be prepared for them not to work after mass events as networks may be overloaded with others trying to make calls.

WHAT WILL I WEAR?

This is probably your most important pre-race planning decision. Deciding what to wear in terms of clothing and on your feet is something that you should do weeks in advance, not on race day. You can then spend time getting used to your racing apparel in training so that there are no nasty surprises on race day. Being fashionable may be great in other areas of life, but marathon clothing is all about comfort and functionality.

TIME TO REFUEL

The final few days are the crucial time for refuelling, so make carbohydrate the main part of your diet and stay properly hydrated. Don't be tempted to overeat, and stick with foods and drinks that you are used to.

WATCH OUT FOR THE WEATHER

Coping with race day weather is possible – controlling it isn't. There are simple measures that can be incorporated into your final preparations so that you are ready for all conditions.

You can control your training, and accumulate the miles that are needed to run a marathon. You can plan meticulously for race day, taper correctly, eat the right foods, and have the perfect race day target time and strategy. But the biggest variable that you can do nothing about is the weather, which can disrupt even the best laid plans and preparation. Having said that, it is possible to reduce the impact of the weather on your performance, and ensure that you have prepared properly for every eventuality.

As we discussed on page 106, most marathons are held in either the spring or autumn, when the weather can vary considerably, and include anything from scorching heat, to the cold and wet. An added problem is that weather conditions can change dramatically throughout the duration of a marathon, with conditions at the start often differing significantly from those at the end. Running in the cold and wet is more of an inconvenience than a thermoregulatory challenge, and there is little that can really be done to prepare for this possibility. But when conditions are hot and humid it makes heat loss less effective, increases the rate of dehydration, running becomes harder, and there is a risk of overheating, or hyperthermia. As we discussed previously, before race day arrives try to find time to train on warmer days – or during the warmest part of the day. This acclimates the body to the heat, and prevents the 'psychological shock' of a hot day, particularly if it is one of the first hot days of the year – a not unusual occurrence when marathons are held in the spring.

Checking the weather forecast in the build up to race day is important, and provides an indication of conditions throughout the race. As well as the

temperature, and whether it could rain, look out for wind conditions too as these can make a huge difference to how you feel. On race day morning, think 'layers', and be prepared to take extra clothes with you that will initially keep you warm during the earlier and colder part of the day, but which can be discarded just before the start of

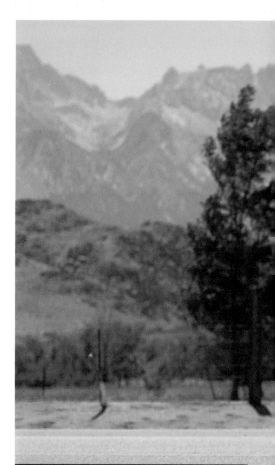

Proper preparation includes checking the race day weather conditions so that you can dress appropriately and prepare mentally.

the race, or even during the early stages as your body temperature increases. Because conditions are often at their coldest at the start, it is all too easy to overdress, and then suffer from being too warm as the race unfolds. Discarding an extra layer, or briefly tolerating the cold in the early stages, is preferable to overdressing and becoming too hot. If it rains before the race, try to keep as dry as possible with either a wet top or bin liner, but once the race starts, it is best to accept that getting wet is inevitable, and if possible keep clothing to a minimum, so that sodden garments are neither heavy nor likely to cause chafing.

If it is warm and sunny on race day, remember that spending many hours in the sunshine running a marathon risks a condition that it is all too easy for runners to overlook – sunburn. Using a high factor sun cream is a very important precaution, and for those who may be lacking a full head of protective hair, a lightweight cap is worthy of consideration.

Coping with variable weather conditions is an inevitable part of marathon running, and doing so successfully ensures that all the hard miles and preparation have the best possible chance of producing a great run. Using the weather to your advantage during training, and adopting a sensible strategy on race day, can all greatly increase your chances of success, regardless of what climatic conditions the race day weather produces.

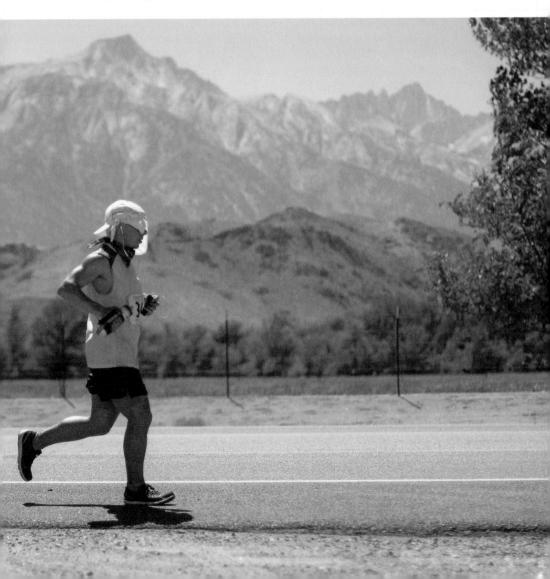

THE LAST FEW HOURS

With race day just around the corner, preparing for the last few hours before the gun goes involves some essential thinking and planning before you finally stand on the start line.

There will come a point, after all the months and weeks of training, when your marathon is just a few hours away. Suddenly it will dominate your mind and everything that you do, inevitably resulting in nervousness and some degree of stress. Knowing how to cope with those final hours, and how to manage your journey to the start line, represents the final part of your marathon preparations.

Packing your bag is one practical aspect of the race that is easy to control. It is best to write out a pre-race check-list and tick each item off, to avoid overlooking something critical. My essential list would always include the following:

- Kit bag
- Race number
- Safety pins
- Running shoes
- Vest or T-shirt, shorts or running tights, and socks
- Petroleum jelly
- Money and phone
- Spare T-shirt/bin liner
- Clothing for the finish
- Snack and drink

These items should be prepared and ready long before you go to bed on pre-race eve. There is nothing worse than a mad panic on race-day morning because a critical item has been forgotten or cannot be found. The spare T-shirt or bin liner are advisable for the start, as a means of keeping warm while standing waiting for the race to begin, but should be disposed of once the race has commenced.

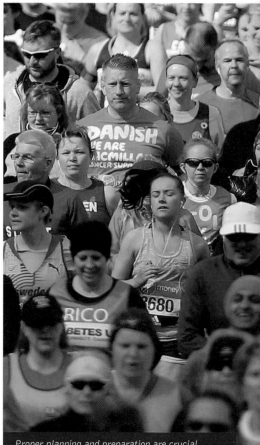
Proper planning and preparation are crucial components of race day success.

It is not uncommon to find runners staying in hotels before a marathon, where the choice of food may differ from what they are used to. This is a time to play it safe, not to experiment with anything exotic or different, while making sure that carbohydrate is a predominant constituent of anything that you eat. Ideally, alcohol should be avoided, or at the very least greatly restricted. It has what is known as

'It is rare for runners to sleep well on the night before a marathon, so while going to bed early may seem sensible, it can often lead to a restless night of sleep. If you find yourself wide awake at 3am worrying about the race ahead, don't worry, you won't be alone.'

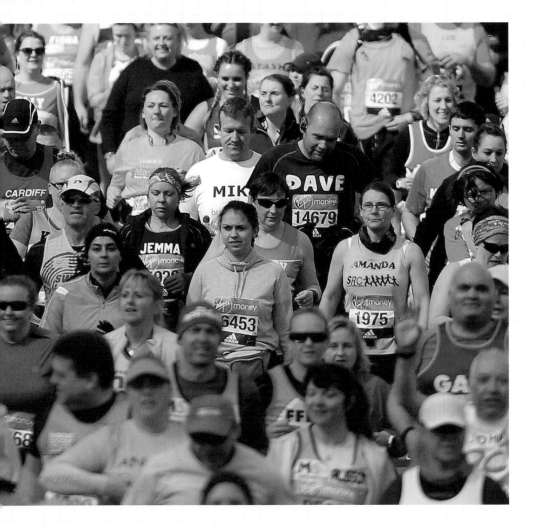

a diuretic effect – it can dehydrate, rather than rehydrate – which is less than ideal, as well as the other negative impacts outlined on page 125.

It is rare for runners to sleep well on the night before a marathon, so while going to bed early may seem sensible, it can often lead to a restless night of sleep. If you find yourself wide awake at 3am worrying about the race ahead, don't worry, you won't be alone! The good news is that while a good night's sleep would be perfect, I have never yet come across a runner who has fallen asleep while running a marathon!

Set your alarm so that you have time for breakfast and don't have to rush to get to the start – it is best to leave extra time rather than to cut things fine, and if you are staying

in an hotel, check to see if they are putting on a breakfast for runners.

Work out your best route to the start, and take snacks and a drink with you – remember that there could be quite a few hours between your breakfast and the start of the race, so staying fuelled and hydrated is important.

When you arrive at the start, check out the toilets and of course make use of them – but be prepared for queues and a functional rather than sweetly perfumed experience. Listen out for final instructions and, when called to do so, head for the start wearing your disposable outer layer, not forgetting to use copious quantities of petroleum jelly to lubricate parts of the body that could rub or chafe.

Finally, focus on the race ahead, revisit your strategy, and get ready for the gun to go.

RACE-DAY PSYCHOLOGY

Marathons play mind games on runners. Coping with nerves and dealing with the mental demands of running 26.2 miles is a key component of race day.

It goes without saying that running a marathon is a huge physical challenge, but the mental approach needed to complete the distance can be equally daunting, and it is all too easy to feel defeated by the task ahead before the race even starts. Coping with and using the nerves and apprehension that are a natural part of race day is essential if the distance is to be completed successfully.

When awaking on the morning of the race, even the most experienced of marathon runners will feel some degree of apprehension; for novices this feeling will be magnified and, if left unchecked, can easily disrupt race-day strategy and performance. At this stage, the most important thing that all runners can and should do is to focus on the positives – you have done the training, you have eaten the right foods, and you have a sensible target and strategy in mind. You can deal with the weather, and you are clear in your mind about the pace you will run at from the outset. Stay completely focussed

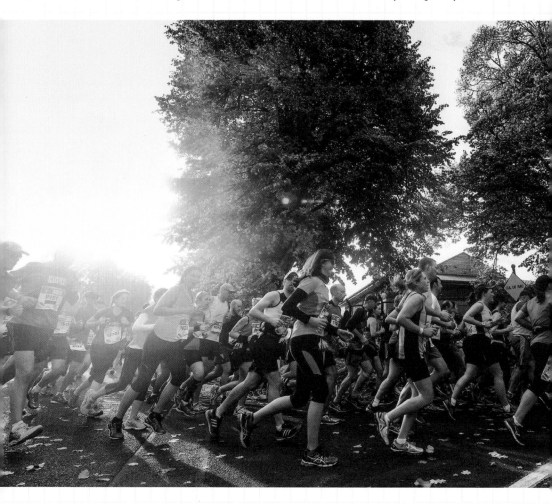

'Staying positive for the first half of the race is crucial. Do not let the distance that is left put you off and keep ticking off 1 mile at a time. Concentrate on what you are achieving, rather than what is to come...'

on these thoughts, and don't let any negative demons into your head. It is common to fall into the trap of thinking 'what am I doing here', 'it's further than I have ever run before' and 'everyone else looks fitter than me'. At this point, it is too late to turn back, and you can guarantee that there will be many other runners all thinking and feeling the same way.

Concentrate on the race ahead, and when the gun goes, avoid the mistake made by so many of setting off too quickly, something

It is all too easy to let the excitement of the day make you forget something critical – like your number!

that is all too easy to do when nervous. In a mass race with lots of other runners, it is not uncommon for the first mile to be congested, and the slowest of the race. This is certainly not the time to panic – there are plenty more miles to come later when time lost at the start can be made up.

Staying positive for the first half of the race is crucial. Do not let the distance that is left put you off and keep ticking off 1 mile at a time. Concentrate on what you are achieving, rather than what is to come, and remind yourself of the all-important 'complete not compete' mantra. Initially, I tend to find that as the miles pass by, the increasing distance that has been run provides a positive endorsement of your running – you feel happy about the miles that you have covered, hopefully while still feeling relatively relaxed and refreshed. One psychological trick that I have tried with some success is to mentally reset the distance that is left once the race has started. This can even be as early as the first mile – just knowing that you no longer have an entire marathon left to run can be a real boost. If your longest training run has been around 20–22 miles, once you reach the 4-mile point, resetting the distance to one that you have already achieved can also give your confidence a big lift.

Quite often in a marathon, there comes a point where instead of focussing on the distance you have covered, your mind is overwhelmed by the distance that is remaining. This frequently coincides with fatigue, and is common at the 16–18-mile point. Suddenly, the 8–10 remaining miles seem an awfully long way. This is the time to dig deep and dispel all negative thoughts. Focus on the finish and concentrate on completing one mile at a time. Forget whether it is the 19th or 23rd mile – just complete each one, then reset for the next. Each mile will pass, and the 26th and final one will eventually arrive.

RACE-DAY NUTRITION

Knowing what to eat - and not to eat - on race day is always a concern. Understanding what and when to eat before and during the race is a key ingredient for success.

No runner needs to eat the energy they need for a marathon on race day – that must come from the diet in the days beforehand. Before the race, it is simply a case of eating what works for you, topping up energy stores, and giving enough time for food in the stomach to be digested before the gun goes. Once the race is underway, personal preferences take over, particularly since the reduction in blood flow to the stomach and intestine makes solid food difficult to digest.

The first – and main – nutritional consideration on race day is the pre-marathon breakfast. I always advise leaving at least 2–3 hours between breakfast and the start of the race, so that food that has been eaten can be properly digested. It is important to eat foods that you have

previous experience of eating prior to running. Carbohydrate foods are of course best – toast, bread, honey, jam, cereals and porridge being common pre-marathon choices. Foods high in fat and protein should be avoided – particularly products such as bacon, sausage and fried eggs. These take time to digest, and provide only a minimal contribution to the type of energy that is needed to run 26.2 miles. Although your next meal is likely to be some time away, it is important to resist the urge to overeat – too much food will take a long time to digest, and could cause stomach problems once the race has started.

I have met many runners who say they are unable to eat breakfast before a race – nerves or just a feeling of nausea afterwards makes this impossible. Although not ideal,

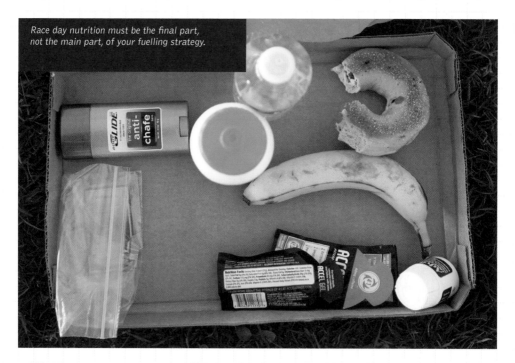

Race day nutrition must be the final part, not the main part, of your fuelling strategy.

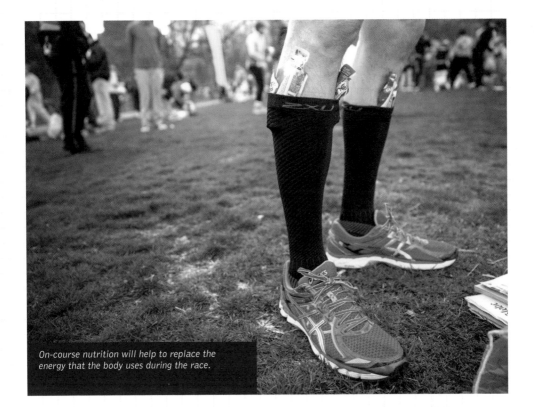

On-course nutrition will help to replace the energy that the body uses during the race.

this is not a disaster, and provided that their nutritional strategy has been correct in the days leading up to the race they should still have high pre-race muscle glycogen stores. As an alternative to solid food, I normally recommend something lighter such as yoghurt or fruit juice, but if even this is not feasible, it is best to let individuals do what is best for them, rather than enforce a perfect scenario that results in a less-than-perfect after-effect!

There may well be a significant period of time between breakfast and the start of the race. I normally recommend that runners take a snack with them to the start, which should again be something familiar that has been tried and tested before running. Bananas are common, as are specially formulated sports energy bars – foods that are high in refined sugar are not advisable too close to the start, since these can cause a rise in insulin levels and increase the rate at which glycogen is used during the early part of the race.

In-race nutrition should again be confined to foods you are comfortable with and have tried before. Some runners take energy foods with them, while many races provide fuel in the form of on-course energy gels. Only take them if you have used them before – what might seem like a good idea at the time could prove to be a big mistake just a few miles later. Similarly, it can often be tempting to accept snacks offered along the course by spectators – despite their well-meaning intentions, I avoid these at all costs. They could be foods that have never been eaten before while running, and a further deterrent is the fact that the hands that are offering them may well have been 'high fiving' sweaty runners just a few minutes earlier. At this stage, risk minimisation is key, and risking a stomach upset when deep into your marathon is not something you want to do.

In short, when it comes to race-day nutrition, following basic scientific principles is important, and performance-inhibiting mistakes should be avoided, but ultimately it is up to each runner to choose what works best for them.

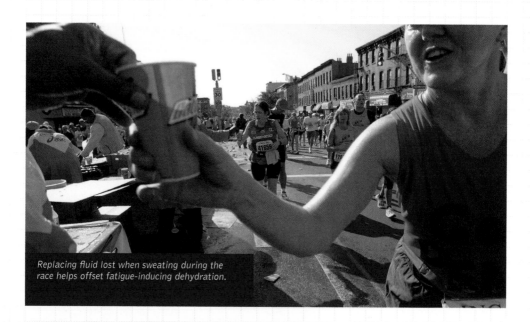

Replacing fluid lost when sweating during the race helps offset fatigue-inducing dehydration.

RACE-DAY HYDRATION

Regardless of the conditions, staying hydrated is important for marathon runners, and a sensible drinking strategy throughout the race will combat the debilitating effects of dehydration.

Regardless of the climate, race-day hydration is critical, since runners will sweat and lose fluid in all conditions. But if the weather is hot and humid, sweat rates will be high, and staying hydrated becomes one of the most important factors influencing performance.

The night before your marathon it is a good idea to sleep with a glass of water by the bedside. Any waking moments during the night can be used as an opportunity to sip some fluid, and when you wake, it is important to rehydrate with around 500ml (17fl oz) of fluid as part of your pre-marathon breakfast. As with nutrition, personal preference is important; some runners prefer coffee or tea, others fruit juice, water or an isotonic drink. Caffeine in coffee has been shown to increase mental alertness, which can be helpful for the start, but the effects will wear off long before the finish! Also be wary about the diuretic effect

of caffeine, since it can produce significant quantities of urine!

Taking fluid on the journey to the start line is also sensible, but at this stage it is important not to overhydrate. Once your urine is clear, you will have rehydrated, and there is no need to overdo it by continually drinking more. The dilemma, of course, is that the more fluid you drink, the more you will need to urinate, which is a common problem faced by many runners (and the owners of adjacent gardens!) during the early stages of a race. It is best to try to target reaching a state of full hydration at least one hour prior to the race start, after which avoid drinking large quantities; sipping small volumes will be sufficient. This should also give time for your bladder to fill and empty, and reduce the chances of a toilet stop early in the race. While water is one means of staying hydrated, isotonic drinks will be absorbed quickly and provide a final top-up of both fluid and energy.

As we have seen on pages 38–39, high sweat rates can soon lead to dehydration in marathon runners, so early use of on-course drinks stations is important, particularly on hot days. Most marathons will provide regular drinks stations for runners – in major events there is often water every mile after the first 3 or 4 miles, and isotonic drinks at less frequent intervals throughout the distance. When added together, these will provide each runner with a significant total volume of fluid, which has the potential to lead to a condition called hyponatremia. This arises when runners drink too much, effectively diluting the body's tissues and inhibiting the function of the muscles and nerves. Along with a risk of nausea and fatigue, in extreme cases hyponatremia can be fatal, so hydrating sensibly is important. Don't be tempted to drink all the fluid that is offered, unless the drink stations are infrequent and conditions are hot. If stations are every mile, then at most half to one-third of a small water bottle should suffice, with

> **'It is often runners towards the back of the field who drink too much - their pace makes it easier to do so, and their sweat rates are often low.'**

sipping and taking small mouthfuls being better than large gulps. It is often runners towards the back of the field who drink too much – their pace makes it easier to do so, and their sweat rates are often low.

The provision of on-course isotonic drinks provides fluid, energy and helps to replace electrolytes lost when sweating. Assuming the brand has been tried previously in training, these are a great and easily absorbed means of topping up energy and, as with energy gels, most will deliver enough energy for around 1 mile of running in a 500ml (17fl oz) bottle – smaller bottles will of course offer less.

Most runners will dehydrate to some extent during a marathon, but minimising this with a sensible hydration strategy before and during the run helps to fight fatigue, maintain sweating and core temperature, and improve performance.

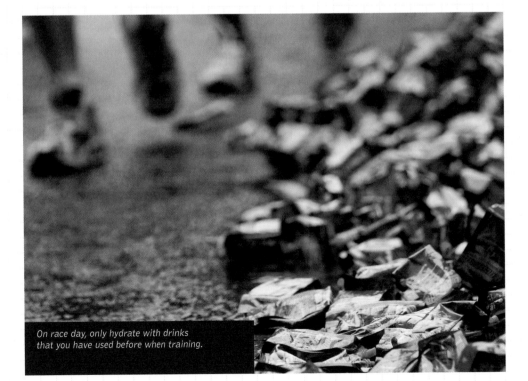

On race day, only hydrate with drinks that you have used before when training.

COPING WITH RACE DAY

Reducing the risks and unknowns that could jeopardise your performance on race day helps to make marathons more about success than unwanted surprises.

In any sport, dealing with the day of competition is crucial, and it is all too easy to undo all the weeks of hard work and dedication through poor preparation and last minute crises. Marathon day is no different – regardless of your goal, knowing what to expect, and how to deal with the unexpected, will help you complete the course successfully.

As already discussed, there are certain things that can be controlled – your waking time, breakfast and journey to the start, along with preparation such as making sure that your kit, number and ancillary items are ready in advance. But there are other variables that runners find harder to control, and things that happen during the race that need to be dealt with. For example, knowing and understanding the course is something that, in my experience, many runners overlook. No one will know every twist and turn of a 26.2-mile route in advance, but it is important to be aware of where the uphill and downhill sections occur, and to mentally

> **'The general euphoria of the early stages of a marathon often leads to runners chanting and 'high fiving' spectators - it may seem boring, but it really is sensible to refrain from anything that expends extra energy.'**

prepare for these ahead of time. Find out where the drinks stations are. Are there are on-course showers or gel stations? If your marathon is overseas, find out whether the distance markers are in miles or kilometres.

The biggest uncontrollable variable is the weather, and checking out the forecast beforehand is crucial. Be prepared for conditions to change as the day and the race unfold, and remember that in general, the coldest time is early in the morning when runners are lining up at the start – once the race begins, heat is generated, and as

the day progresses, the temperature will probably rise.

The very nature of mass-participation marathons entails lining up on the start with many other runners. It is therefore not a surprise that when the start gun sounds, for many, nothing happens. At some point everyone will begin to shuffle forwards, then walk, jog and eventually run – a process that often means it takes many minutes to even reach the start line. It is important not to panic! In many races, personal-timing chips

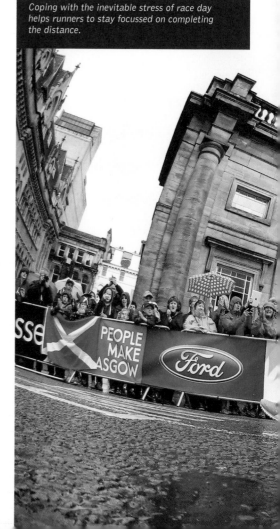

Coping with the inevitable stress of race day helps runners to stay focussed on completing the distance.

will be issued to all runners so that each individual's race time only begins once the start line has been crossed. Furthermore, as we have discussed, starting slowly is beneficial as it uses less muscle glycogen, and there is still more than enough distance left to make up for any time lost at the start.

Once the race is underway, there will inevitably be runners trying to push their way past in an attempt to get towards the front. Don't be tempted to copy them, and try to find space where the risk of a trip or heavy fall is minimised. The general euphoria of the early stages of a marathon often leads to runners chanting and 'high fiving' spectators – it may seem boring, but it really is sensible to refrain from anything that expends extra energy. This is a time to stay relaxed, settle into a rhythm and your pace, and to focus on the task ahead.

As the race unfolds, the different sights, sounds, topography and climate will change the nature of the event. Family and friends may be at prearranged points to give a psychological boost, but it is all too easy to miss them in major races where the crowds are plentiful. In lower-key events, be prepared for long miles of loneliness, with few others around, until you finally approach the finish line. When you cross that line, you will temporarily be lighter (mainly through a loss of body fluid), and shorter – the constant impact with the ground will have compressed your spine. But you will have completed the distance and run a marathon, and coped with a day and event that will be one of the few moments in your life that will always be remembered.

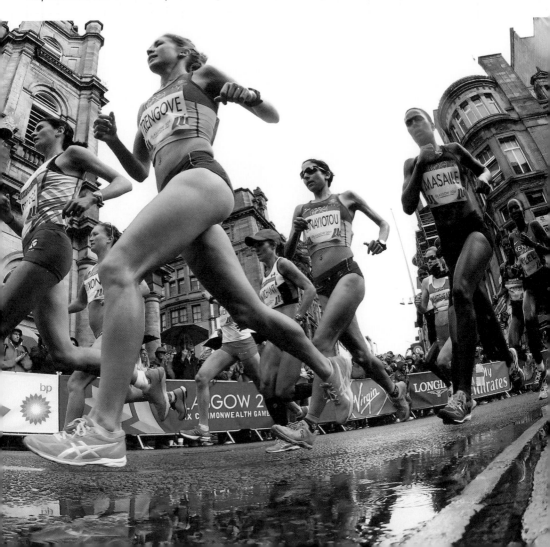

MYTH: *YOU MUST USE CARBO GELS*

Carbo gels are a relatively recent addition to the sports nutrition cupboard, and have been designed to provide a concentrated burst of carbohydrate in a small, easy-to-carry sachet. Their use has increased in endurance events since they are conveniently transported in a running belt or shorts pocket, and because they are offered on-course at many of the major marathon events.

Carbo gels come in a range of sizes, and tend to have a thick 'gloopy' texture that is somewhere between that of a liquid and a jelly. Most contain around 30g (11/2oz) of carbohydrate, or 120kcal of energy, which is enough for most runners to run 1 mile. But of course, that doesn't mean that runners need to take 26 of them when completing a marathon. The body's existing

stores of carbohydrate, in addition to energy from fat, mean that it should be possible to reach way beyond the 20-mile point before you need an energy boost from a gel. This means, provided they have been tried before the race, that with good training, pacing and pre-race nutrition, eating one or two gels during a marathon should be sufficient.

Gels are especially beneficial towards the end of a race, and have helped many marathon runners to overcome the last few tough miles, by providing energy from their calories, and a psychological boost from their sweet taste. But they are not essential – many hundreds of thousands of marathon runners successfully completed marathons long before carbo gels were ever invented – and marathons can and will continue to be completed successfully without them.

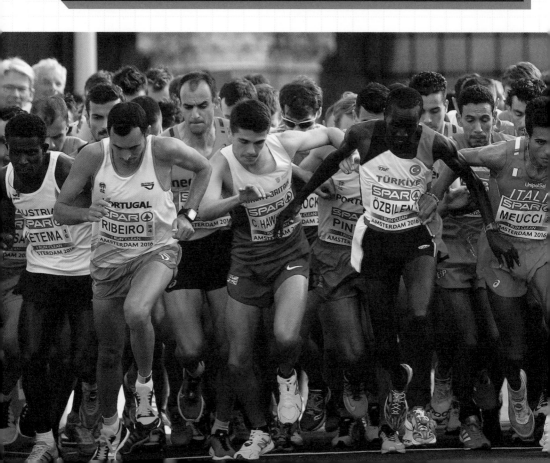

MYTH: *I NEED A GOOD START TO GET A GOOD TIME*

There are times when the start of a marathon more closely resembles a rugby match than an endurance event, especially in mass events with many thousands of runners lining up along the length and width of narrow streets. For those not on or close to the start line, there is frequently a disappointing lack of movement when the start gun sounds, and this is quickly replaced by alarm as the seconds and even minutes tick by. Runners who feel trapped and slowed by those in front try to push and side-step their way forwards, often endangering their own progress in the race and that of those around them.

However, in the vast majority of cases, starting slowly really does not matter, and can actually be a benefit in the latter stages. Marathons are endurance events,

not sprints, and there are plenty of minutes and miles ahead to regain time lost at the start. Furthermore, starting slowly helps to spare carbohydrate stores by enabling the muscles to burn more fat, and this will leave more carbohydrate to provide you with energy towards the end of the race. Most races will have pens or zones where runners can line up at the start in an order based on their predicted finishing time. It really is important to adhere to these since it prevents slower runners blocking the path of those running more quickly and lessens the chance of running alongside others at a pace that is too quick.

So start slowly, stay relaxed and don't panic if your first few miles are slower than planned, and leave plenty in reserve for the final push to the finish line.

The start is a time of high excitement and high risk, so the emphasis must be to start sensibly and safely.

RACE-DAY STRATEGY

Marathons make you tired, no matter how fit you are and how fast you run. Help is at hand, however, and having a strategy to cope with running 26.2 miles is one of the best ways of managing marathon fatigue.

Standing on the start line, with not only a realistic target time but also a pacing strategy with which to achieve it, is one of the most important components of marathon success. Having the discipline to stick with the strategy throughout the race, however, is a challenge, but doing so can make marathons much more achievable.

This is not always easy if others around you are running at a pace faster than yours should be, so in events where runners line up in starting pens according to ability and

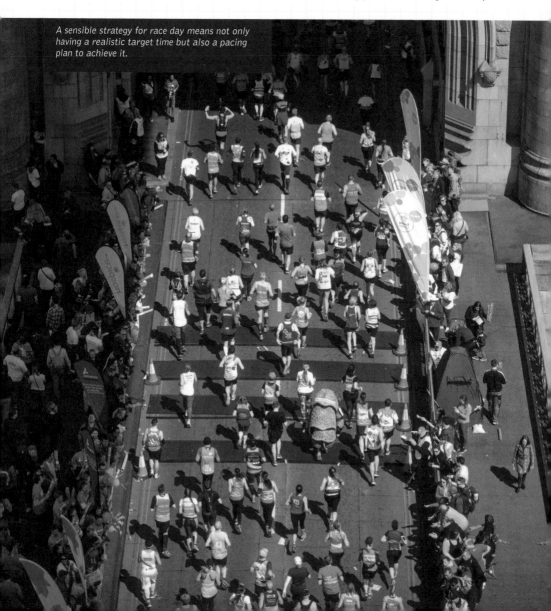

A sensible strategy for race day means not only having a realistic target time but also a pacing plan to achieve it.

MYTH: *NASAL STRIPS WILL HELP ME TO BREATHE*

Small strips of plastic, originally designed to help cure snoring, have become a frequent feature on the faces of many runners. Stretching from one side of the lower nose to the other and sticking to the outside of each nostril, they pull the nostrils open, widening their diameter so that, in theory, the entry of air into the nose – and ultimately the lungs – becomes easier.

However, once running starts, the genuine benefit of nasal strips is negligible. The human body can use two routes to get air into the lungs – through the mouth (oral breathing), or through the nose (nasal breathing). A combination of the two can also be used – a process perhaps not surprisingly known as 'oral-nasal' breathing. Nasal breathing filters and warms the air before it enters the lungs,

something that breathing orally fails to do. However, scientific studies have shown that when we move from rest to exercise and the demand for air increases rapidly, the narrower passageways of the nose, even when using nasal strips, increases resistance and makes it difficult, if not impossible, to obtain the desired volume of air nasally. Consequently, at anything more than modest ventilation rates, we subconsciously choose to breath orally, and this is the most common and efficient method of breathing when marathon running, even if nasal strips are worn.

Nasal strips may enable runners to use oral-nasal breathing for longer before resorting to oral breathing, but nasal breathing, with or without a nasal strip, is highly unlikely to be the preferred method of breathing for marathon runners.

---

predicted finish time, it is important to choose the right position, and to start with others aiming for a similar pace and time. After possible congestion at the start, the first few miles are a time to settle into your desired pace. It may be the third or fourth mile before this becomes possible but, once achieved, this is when you should relax, reduce energy expenditure and, when the first drink station occurs, start to replace fluid that will have already been lost. Most runners feel the occasional twinge and ache when running, and the first few miles of a marathon are no exception. It is all too easy to over-emphasise these and panic, but in the vast majority of cases they are no different to those that happen when training, and will soon go or be forgotten about as the race unfolds. Making a conscious effort to relax the arms and shoulders, to breathe in a relaxed manner and, if there are spectators, using their encouragement for motivation, should all help to make the early miles ones

'Although the mathematical mid-point of a marathon is 13.1 miles, most experienced runners will say that in terms of effort, the second half really only begins at around 16-18 miles.'

of minimal effort and maximal relaxation.

You should aim to reach the halfway point feeling as good as possible, and at your pre-planned pace and target time. Although the mathematical mid-point of a marathon is 13.1 miles, most experienced runners will say that in terms of effort, the second half really only begins at around 16–18 miles. Consequently, the miles from 13 to 18 are, in my experience, all important. They mark the transition from the mid-point to the latter stages of the race, and keeping your pacing on track, managing the symptoms of fatigue, and staying mentally focussed and positive, will help to get you to the final part of the race in a much better physical and psychological shape. Of course there will be inevitable chafing from constant rubbing, and twinges from your feet that may signal a blister or the imminent departure of a toenail or two, but these can be ignored and dealt with once the race is over.

As the 20-mile mark is reached, some degree of dehydration and depletion of muscle-glycogen stores is certainly going to result in fatigue, and each stride will become harder. The use of on-course fluid and energy provision helps to mitigate this, and makes the final miles more tolerable. Psychologically, this is a time to concentrate

'**If all is going to plan, and the strategy and pacing are on track, the inevitable fatigue of the last few miles will be overcome by focussing on the achievement of your goal.**'

on the distance that has been achieved, and not become subsumed by the distance that is still to come. If all is going to plan, and the strategy and pacing are on track, the inevitable fatigue of the last few miles will be overcome by focussing on the achievement of your goal, and the need not to lose time by slowing down with the finish line in sight.

As fatigue builds, simple tactics such as a slight change in stride length may help to unlock reserves of glycogen in different muscle fibres, and simply tasting something sweet, even if not actually consuming anything, may give a short-term performance boost. Avoid slumping forwards as tiredness builds, since this can make breathing harder. Run tall, keep your form and pace, and the finish will soon arrive. By digging deep, you may even make the final couple of miles your fastest of the race!

MYTH: *A STITCH MEANS STOPPING*

It's easy to forget that during a marathon the muscles used to support breathing – the respiratory muscles – have a lot in common with the leg muscles; they need to do a lot of hard and continuous work. Between 8000 and 10,000 breaths transport around 25,000 litres (44,000 pints) of air into and out of the lungs when running 26.2 miles, and this means a lot of effort for the respiratory muscles that lift and lower the ribcage, and the diaphragm muscle lying just beneath the ribcage, which helps to draw air into the lungs.

So it's not a surprise that at times these muscles also succumb to the rigours of a marathon. 'Stitch' is the term given to a sudden inability to breathe deeply, often accompanied by tightening and pain in the lower part of the lungs and ribcage. The exact causes of stitch are not really

understood – it could simply be fatigue and cramping of the diaphragm, perhaps as a reaction to cold air entering the lungs, or cold fluid entering the stomach. The effects of a stitch are normally quite short-lived, and although for a time it can cause a runner to slow or even stop, in most cases it can be overcome. Gently stretching by bending towards the opposite side of the stitch, or slowly breathing deeply to stretch the respiratory muscles and diaphragm, can help to relieve the symptoms, and running can be resumed – slowly at first – once they have passed. As with any problem, prevention is better than cure; sipping drinks rather than gulping and occasionally taking long, deep breaths to relax the respiratory muscles helps to prevent a problem that is inconvenient rather than race-ending.

MYTH: *YOU CAN'T WALK AND MANAGE A GOOD MARATHON TIME*

When most people go for a steady walk, they cover the ground at around 3 miles per hour, taking 20 minutes to complete each mile. Multiply this by 26.2, and it equates to finishing a marathon in 8 hours and 44 minutes. That is not a fast marathon time by any stretch of the imagination, and in many major marathons it would mean finishing outside of the cut-off time, with no official time, medal, or the all-important finisher's T-shirt.

However, increase the pace just a bit, and it can start to make a huge difference to the final time. For many of us, brisk walking equates to around 4 miles per hour (15 minutes per mile), whereas a steady jog is closer to 10–11 minutes per mile. So including a mixture of running,

jogging, brisk and steady walking can quickly – and relatively easily – result in an average pace of 15 minutes per mile or even less. At 15 minutes per mile pace, a marathon will be completed in just over 6 hours 30 minutes, while an average pace of 12 minutes per mile – which could be achieved with a combination of running and walking – results in a respectable finishing time of just outside 5 hours.

In conclusion, while having to walk makes winning a marathon very tricky, if not impossible, walking can form part of a successful strategy that has finishing the distance as the main objective. Moreover, if it is combined with a reasonable amount of running, walking will also result in a respectable finishing time.

MYTH: *FASTER RUNNING BURNS MORE CALORIES THAN SLOW RUNNING*

It is a common misconception to assume that if you complete a training run or a marathon quickly, you will burn more calories than if you cover the same distance slowly. In fact, while the rate of energy burn will be higher when running fast, the total number of calories used to get from the start to the end of the run will be pretty much the same, regardless of running speed. Moving a fixed mass from one point to another will, on the whole, require a fairly constant amount of energy – it is just that fast running often feels as if it should be burning more total calories, since it requires greater effort. However, that effort ends sooner than it does when you are running more slowly, so eventually the longer, slower calorie burn matches the

energy used when running the same distance more quickly.

Running economy – the amount of energy used to run a set distance – does vary slightly between runners, often as a result of differences in experience, style and bodyweight. There will also be some individual fluctuation for the same runner, caused by differences in efficiency when running at slower or faster speeds. But these differences are surprisingly small, and as a consequence it is possible to estimate the amount of energy that runners use for specific distances. For example, most runners will burn around 100–120 calories to run a single mile, regardless of speed, and will burn a total of around 3000 calories running a marathon, whether in 2 hours or 5 hours.

Optimising your marathon recovery strategy makes the return to full fitness quicker, and less painful.

SECTION FOUR
MARATHON RECOVERY

The marathon has been run and your body has undergone immense stresses. Marathon recovery is just as important as marathon preparation and this section explains the optimal ways to recover and how to return to normal post-marathon life.

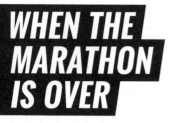

WHEN THE MARATHON IS OVER

For most runners, crossing the finish line brings euphoria and an end to the 26.2-mile challenge. For some, failing to finish will bring disappointment. Dealing with both and moving on is the next priority.

For months you will have prepared and focussed on your marathon. It will have dominated your life, and that of those closest to you. Then, after you have crossed the finish line, it is all over, and time to return to normality, at least for a while, or until the next challenge. This is when the process of recovery becomes an important part of marathon running; neglecting it could make the journey back to normal life, or running again, much longer and harder.

For most marathon runners the recovery process will take place alongside a prolonged 'runners high' and feeling of euphoria – a desire to tell everyone about your achievement, and to wear your medal continuously for many days to come. For a small minority though, there will be disappointment, either as a result of failing to achieve a desired time or, worse still, through a failure to finish. In my experience, any disappointment with a slower-than-expected time quickly fades – after all the distance has still been accomplished, and 26.2 miles is a long and tough distance to cover, regardless of running speed. Failing to finish is different, and can be a devastating blow when the marathon has been the

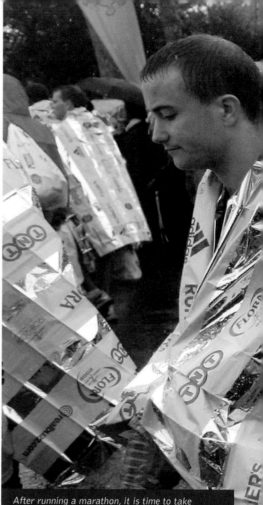

After running a marathon, it is time to take stock, reflect on your achievement and decide what to do next.

culmination of many miles of long and lonely training. There is no easy or quick solution to this, and the nature of the failure will impact on how long the recovery stage takes. If it was simply down to fatigue, then after a few weeks of mental and physical recovery, attempting another marathon is an option. But if it happened as a result of injury, then the process of rehabilitation and recovery could be much longer. That said, even runners who fail to finish will have developed a significant amount of 'marathon fitness', and this can still be utilised to prepare for another attempt at the distance if the desire to try again remains.

The short-term aftermath of finishing a marathon is all about getting your medal, goodie bag and finisher's T-shirt, then being

> **'The process of recovery becomes an important part of marathon running; neglecting it could make the journey back to normal life, or running again, much longer and harder.'**

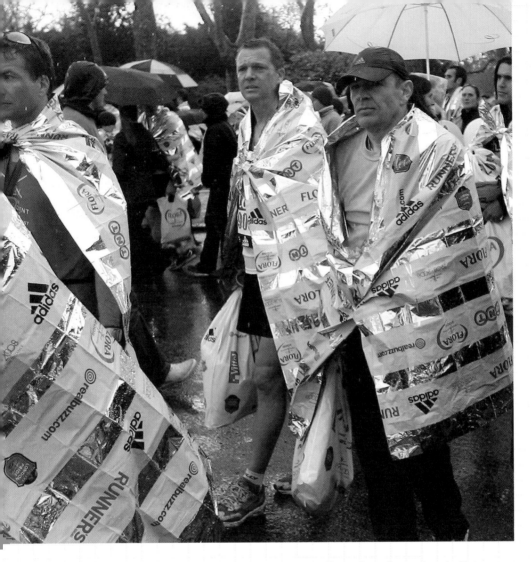

reunited with your kit bag, friends and family. This can take some time, and keeping warm is a high priority. As soon as running stops, heart rate and the demand for oxygen will decrease. Less blood will reach the leg muscles, and as they are no longer producing heat, body temperature will soon start to drop, which can quickly result in shivering. As a result, many races will provide lightweight 'space blankets' for finishers, which should be used to retain body heat.

All marathons will have a system in place to help runners find their kit, and in races where the start and finish are in different locations, clothing will have been transported to the finish in baggage buses. Finding your baggage bus and bag is normally a relatively quick and efficient process. Once you have done so, it is the time to change out of your running kit, put on extra layers, and start the all-important process of rehydrating and refuelling.

Locating family and friends can be tricky unless a meeting point has been prearranged, and never underestimate the chaos caused by crowds and other runners all intent on doing the same thing. At major events, phone networks may be overloaded, so planning and patience are crucial. There may well be a designated meeting area, with easily identified letters or numbers that can be used as meeting locations. For weary runners, it is often easiest to find a spot in which to wait and let others do the finding!

PRACTICAL STEPS FOR RECOVERY

There is life after a marathon, but it takes time to recover and return to normal. Simple self-help steps will help to make the recovery process quick and effective.

When the marathon is over, recovery starts. Of course you will eventually recover if you do nothing, but it could be a long – and at times painful – process. Taking the simple steps outlined below to aid recovery will help marathon runners of all abilities return to normal quickly and effectively.

REHYDRATE
Use non-alcoholic fluids such as an isotonic drink to replace fluid, fuel and electrolytes.

REFUEL
You will have used close to the equivalent of a full day's energy intake, and glycogen stores will be depleted, so carbohydrates must be a central part of your diet during the days after the race.

BLISTERS, CHAFING AND LOST TOENAILS
These are inevitable, and if serious, may need cleaning, disinfecting and strapping by a medical expert. If they aren't too bad, keep damaged areas clean, dry and covered until they heal.

DOMS
Delayed Onset Muscle Soreness or DOMS is the term that refers to the most common – and in most runners' experience the most painful – post-marathon symptom. DOMS is caused by damage and inflammation of the muscle fibres and surrounding tissue as a result of the continuous impact on the road. This builds to a peak 24–48 hours after the marathon is over, hence the use of the word 'delayed', and can be quite debilitating when at its most severe, making walking difficult, especially when walking downhill or down stairs. For many, DOMS is a 'badge of honour' and sends a clear signal to more sedentary friends that you have just run a marathon! DOMS is

temporary, but some relief can be obtained by having a warm bath, which relaxes the muscles and helps to remove the build-up of fluid and inflammation that is causing the soreness.

ICE BATHS
These have become popular with runners, especially elite ones, as a means of reducing the inflammation that leads to muscle soreness and DOMS. They should occur during the first few hours after a marathon, which can present practical problems for those faced with a long journey home. For many, having endured the pain associated with running 26.2 miles, further discomfort in a bath of ice is not overly endearing. View it as an optional post-race extra for the hardy, rather than a 'must do'!

STRETCHING
Gentle stretching of the muscles that have worked hard will help to reduce muscle stiffness and inflammation, and stimulate blood flow to aid healing and recovery.

MASSAGE
There are differing opinions on the benefits of a post-marathon massage. Immediately after the race it is important not to further aggravate damaged muscles with a deep massage, although gentle massage may help to stimulate blood flow and reduce stiffness. Many runners prefer to book a massage for two or three days after their marathon, when the recovery process is well underway and the muscles can more easily be manipulated. At this point, a massage can help to reduce inflammation and relax the muscles, making it easier for normal muscle contractions to resume. Using rollers to gently massage sore muscles after a marathon is popular, and may help to relax muscles and increase blood flow to prevent and reduce stiffness.

RUNNING

When to run again after a marathon depends very much on each individual, and how much physiological and psychological stress the event has caused. For most people, running should be possible within a week, but this should be slow and over a relatively short distance. Be prepared for the legs to feel tired, especially at the start.

WHAT NEXT?

Set a new goal. Is it another marathon, something shorter such as a 10km race, or an even greater goal such as an ultra-endurance event or a triathlon? It is worth remembering that running and training for a marathon will result in significant improvements in fitness, so as recovery progresses, using this fitness again, rather than losing it, is an attractive option.

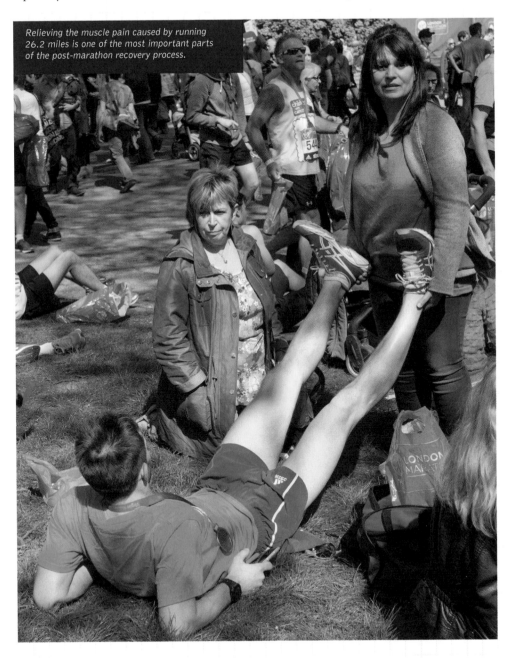

Relieving the muscle pain caused by running 26.2 miles is one of the most important parts of the post-marathon recovery process.

Many events present unusual physiological and mental demands and prove a challenge for even the most experienced marathon runners.

NEW CHALLENGES

After months of hard work and dedication you have joined the esteemed club of marathon finishers. For many this will be just the beginning, since there are numerous other marathon events and challenges to tackle.

WHAT NEXT?

Completing 26.2 miles can be the start, rather than the end, of a life-changing process. Setting new goals and targets, rather than waiting for all that hard-earned fitness to be lost, is a great next step once the marathon is over.

When it's all over, and you have crossed the finishing line, it is likely that the first words you will say are 'never again'. But for many, when the pain has subsided and been replaced by the warm glow of success and pride, it doesn't take long to start contemplating the next challenge. This does not need to be another marathon – there are plenty of races over much shorter and easier distances that can be completed regularly and with much less effort and lifestyle change. These include 5km, 10km, 10 miles and half-marathon races, which are held regularly in venues across many countries, and provide a chance to stay fit and healthy while enjoying the camaraderie of competition. Individuals who have completed a marathon will have developed a high level of fitness that will become apparent once the process of physical and mental recovery has been completed. To lose this fitness by doing nothing would be a great shame, whereas capitalising on it to enter new events and set different goals is likely to bring significant lifestyle and health benefits.

For some, completing another marathon becomes the next goal, perhaps in a faster time, or in a different part of the country or even the world. Some runners become 'marathon tourists', choosing cities and countries to visit where marathons are held, combining their running with holidays and using their marathon as an excuse to sightsee rather than as an attempt to run a personal-best time. Today, nearly every major capital city in the world has its own marathon, while others, such as the Everest Marathon, offer the chance to take part in what are often more challenging events in extreme or unusual locations.

The choice of alternatives for runners who have completed a marathon is far greater than it was even 20 years ago. Ultra-marathons offer the chance to complete distances in excess of 26.2 miles, and provide a real challenge for those for whom marathon running is simply not hard enough! But as well as these and the numerous shorter events held in the countryside, towns and cities each weekend, there are also multi-discipline events such as triathlons and duathlons.

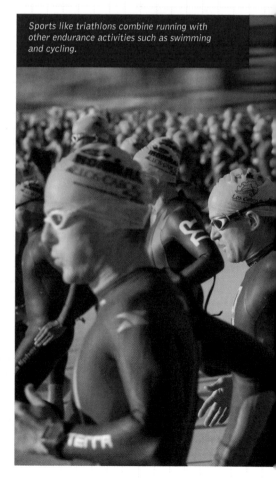

Sports like triathlons combine running with other endurance activities such as swimming and cycling.

Triathlons have grown rapidly in popularity – once thought of as the domain of extreme endurance athletes, today triathlons (swimming, cycling and running) have become accessible to many more people with a range of abilities, who can swim, cycle and run over either long 'iron man' distances, or take part in shorter 'sprint' events. For those who find swimming the hardest of the triathlon disciplines, duathlons – a combination of cycling and running – have also become increasingly popular.

There is no doubt that running a marathon transforms many lives. As we have discovered, this is most evident in the build-up to the race, when the training and dedication that are required can take over the lives of the runners and their families. But if used to good effect, the completion of a marathon can also transform lives for

'Ultra-marathons offer the chance to train and complete over distances in excess of 26.2 miles, and provide a real challenge for those for whom marathon running is simply not hard enough!'

many years after the race has been completed. Embedding exercise into our routine and constantly setting and working towards goals helps people to lead more active lives, and to make societies healthier. If you only ever run one marathon in your life, but use the experience to make exercise a regular part of all that you do, then the benefits will last for many years to come. But if you choose to run multiple marathons, or set challenges and targets that require levels of mental and physical endurance that go beyond those needed to run 26.2 miles, then the opportunities are almost endless.

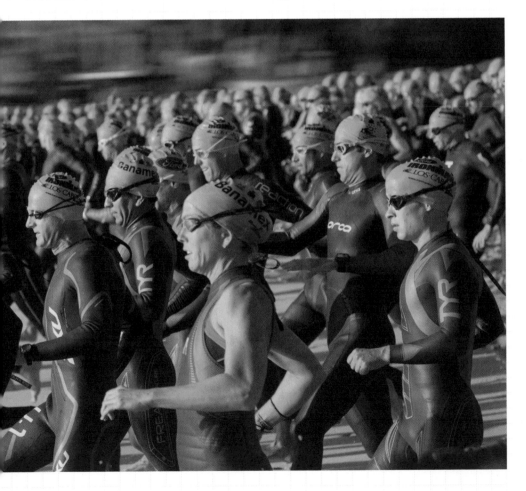

THE MARATHON MAJORS

The high-profile, big-city, mass-participation Marathon Majors attract runners from all over the world, and finishing each of them at least once has become a 'must-do' target for many runners.

The 'Majors' is a series of six marathons held annually around the world – Boston, Berlin, Chicago, London, New York and Tokyo. They are all big-city, mass-participation events, and must comply with the highest standards of administration and organisation, as well as giving a proven commitment to anti-doping. For elite runners, the Majors offer a chance to win substantial prize money, with points scored for the best performances in any two of the races, which are totalled to determine an annual winner. The organisers of each Major will frequently use science to support their runners, which includes advice on pre-race preparation, nutrition and training, as well as on-course hydration and post-race recovery strategies. To avoid extremes of climate, the Majors are held during either the spring or autumn months, although in 2012 the New York Marathon had to be cancelled as a result of a hurricane. The high profile of each race attracts runners from overseas, and for many, the challenge of overcoming jet lag and resetting their circadian rhythms can make running 26.2 miles even harder than normal!

BOSTON, USA

Always held on Patriots Day, the third Monday in April, Boston is the world's oldest annual marathon, having first been run in 1897. Runners must achieve a qualifying time to take part, and the race is known for its tough series of hills, culminating in 'Heartbreak Hill' between 20 and 21 miles. Although Heartbreak Hill only climbs 21m

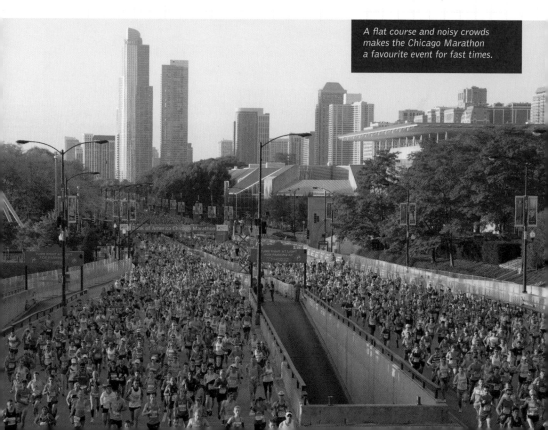

A flat course and noisy crowds makes the Chicago Marathon a favourite event for fast times.

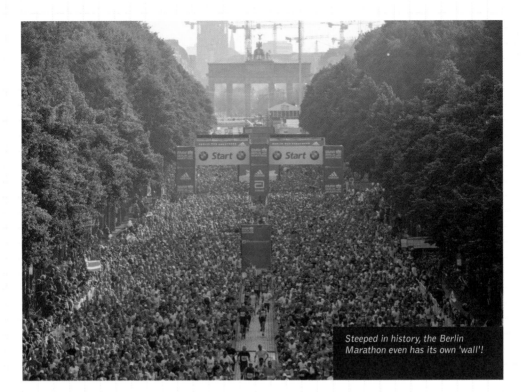

Steeped in history, the Berlin Marathon even has its own 'wall'!

(88ft), its reputation comes from its location at the point where glycogen stores are close to depletion.

BERLIN, GERMANY

Held in September, the Berlin Marathon starts and finishes near the iconic Brandenburg Gate (see photo, above). The course changed in 1990 when the reunification of Germany enabled it to cover all of Berlin, and every runner has a close encounter with the remains of the Berlin Wall at the 24-mile point.

CHICAGO, USA

Attracting around 1.7 million spectators and passing through 29 neighbourhoods, the Chicago Marathon is held in October and has seen many world records. The flat course, noise from the crowds, and a limited number of twists and turns all contribute to making the event conducive to fast times (see photo, left).

LONDON, UK

The London Marathon is held in April, with simultaneous starts in Greenwich and Blackheath. Runners take in many of London's greatest sights before finishing on The Mall in front of Buckingham Palace. The slight downhill section for the first 3 miles can lure runners into starting too quickly, but thereafter the course is flat with frequent hydration and refuelling stations.

NEW YORK, USA

The largest marathon in the world, with over 50,000 finishers, the New York Marathon passes through the five boroughs of New York City. It has been held each year since 1970, apart from 2012, when it was cancelled as a result of the impact of Hurricane Sandy.

TOKYO, JAPAN

With a course that combines historic and modern parts of the city, the Tokyo Marathon attracts around 35,000 runners when it is held in February each year. It is the largest marathon in Asia and is likely to include parts of the route that will be used for the Olympic Games' marathon in 2020.

MARATHONS MADE FOR SCIENTISTS

All marathons are tough, but some are just that little bit tougher, with their location or climate providing runners with an extra level of difficulty that makes them stand out from the rest.

While the 26.2 miles of any marathon will always provide a challenge to the human body, there are others that stretch the boundaries of human performance just a little bit further, and it is in these that science can make even more of an impact if applied properly.

THE EVEREST MARATHON, NEPAL

Starting close to Everest Base Camp, at an altitude of 5184m (17,000ft) (see photo, right), the rarefied atmosphere and reduced oxygen content of the Everest Marathon mean that acclimatisation to running at high altitude is essential. The race is largely downhill, finishing in the Sherpa village of Namche Bazaar, at a still-demanding altitude of 3446m (11,300ft). Downhill running over difficult terrain involves plenty of eccentric contractions to induce muscle soreness, which can make post-marathon recovery a long and painful process.

THE DEATH VALLEY MARATHON, CALIFORNIA, USA

Unlike the Everest Marathon, this race is held entirely below sea level in the spectacular setting of the floor of Death Valley, one of the hottest places on the planet. Temperatures often reach 30–40°C (86–104°F), making dehydration and hyperthermia a constant threat. Acclimation to running in hot conditions is an essential prerequisite for all competitors if they are to complete the distance safely and successfully.

THE NORTH POLE MARATHON, THE NORTH POLE

Overheating is not a problem with this marathon, but keeping warm is. Held on a 26.2-mile course inside the Arctic Circle and close to the North Pole, the route varies from year to year depending on the ice conditions. This race often involves conditions of extreme cold, which means that running in thermal

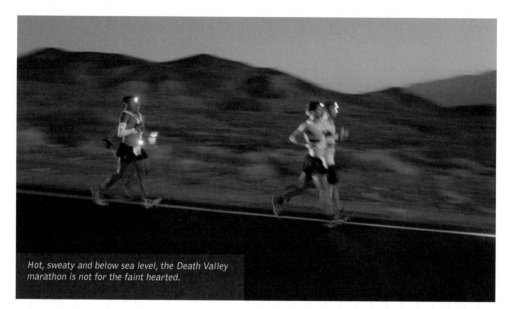

Hot, sweaty and below sea level, the Death Valley marathon is not for the faint hearted.

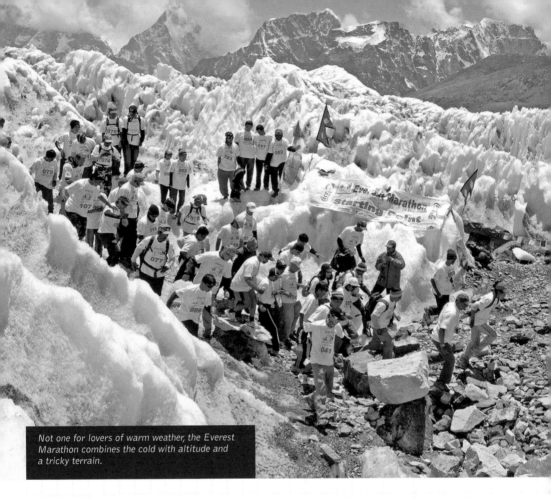

Not one for lovers of warm weather, the Everest Marathon combines the cold with altitude and a tricky terrain.

clothing, and keeping the extremities covered to prevent frostbite, is essential. The cold can be a particular problem for runners who fatigue and slow down, since they consequently stop generating the heat needed to maintain core temperature.

NORTH DORSET VILLAGES MARATHON, UK

Not every marathon is a mass-participation, big-city event, or one that is held in extreme conditions. There are plenty more where the entry fields are small, and spectators are sparse. These inevitably result in long stretches of lonely running where self-motivation is critical, testing psychological resilience as well as physical capacity and reserves. The North Dorset Villages Marathon is one such event, with a small entry field, a friendly atmosphere and a rural route that runs through a series of picturesque villages in North Dorset. Post-race nutrition comes courtesy of a hog roast, along with a vegetarian alternative. This is a race for those who want to get away from the crowds, rely on mental toughness, and engage with the countryside rather than the noise, bustle and concrete of a big-city event.

THE MEDOC MARATHON

The Medoc Marathon breaks every rule and scientific theory of marathon running. Held in Bordeaux, France, fancy dress is compulsory, and at each of the 23 refuelling stops, runners are expected to drink a glass of wine while partaking in local delicacies such as oysters, foie gras and cheese. Not a race for the faint-hearted or for those with a delicate stomach, the Medoc Marathon attracts 10,000 runners each year, with a cut-off time for reaching – or staggering over – the finishing line of 6 hours 30 minutes.

ULTRA-MARATHONS

Some runners looking for their next challenge after a marathon enter a 5km race. Others decide on something more extreme, such as an ultra-marathon, which tests endurance over distances well beyond 26.2 miles.

If running 26.2 miles no longer seems far enough, ultra-marathons provide a chance to run longer and further, placing additional mental and physical stresses on the body.

After completing a first marathon, for some runners that is it, and never again will the same distance be attempted. For others, it may mark the start of more marathons and, perhaps a desire to run even further to test the limits of personal endurance. As a result, ultra-marathons – defined as any distance beyond the 26.2 miles of the marathon – have grown in popularity as more and more runners who have become accomplished at marathons seek out new challenges.

There are two types of ultra-marathon: the first is time based, where runners aim to cover as much distance as possible in a set time, such as 24 or 48 hours. The second – and most common – is based on distance where, as with any race, the aim is to cover a set distance as quickly as possible. No ultra-marathon is ever going to be 'easy', but the distance that is the closest extension of the marathon is 50km (31 miles), and provides a good entry point for those who are new to ultras. Beyond this, distances such as 100km (62 miles) and 100 miles are common, sometimes held on roads or at cross-country, multi-terrain routes, or around athletic tracks. Before entering any ultra, it is important to undertake some background research, and check on the support that is offered, the terrain (and possible hills!), and whether navigation skills are needed.

Extreme ultras provide an ultimate challenge; the infamous Tour du Mont Blanc starts and finishes in Chamonix each August and competitors have 48 hours to complete 164km (102 miles) of mountain running through France, Italy and Switzerland, climbing and descending over 8000m (26,250ft) before crossing the finish line – almost the equivalent of climbing and descending Mount Everest!

MYTH: *TAKING SALT CURES CRAMP*

One minute, all is going well, with each stride slowly ticking off the miles. Then in an instant, the burning, crippling tightening of a muscle turns a fluid runner into a stumbling wreck. Muscle cramping can be debilitating and devastating, and occurs out of the blue or, for some runners, is a regular affliction that they have to cope with.

The exact cause of cramp is not fully understood, and may vary from one person to another. The muscles are placed under heavy, repetitive stress during a marathon, within an environment that is constantly changing. Billions of coordinated nerve impulses trigger muscle fibres to produce energy via a highly complex biochemical process, which causes muscle to contract and relax many thousands of times. This takes place in an environment that is constantly changing.

One possible theory behind the cause of cramp is the fact that sweating causes the loss of electrolytes – particularly sodium – which are needed to support muscle and nerve function. Since sodium is a form of salt, some runners take salt tablets in an attempt to minimise the risk of cramp. This is a mistake, since as running progresses, the concentration of sodium within the body actually increases, despite the loss of some in sweat. This is because proportionally, fluid is lost at a greater rate, so while the total amount of sodium within the body drops, the concentration within body fluids actually increases. Taking salt tablets will increase the concentration even further, and potentially make the problem far worse. Staying hydrated, using an isotonic drink that replaces fluid and electrolytes, and stretching, are more sensible options.

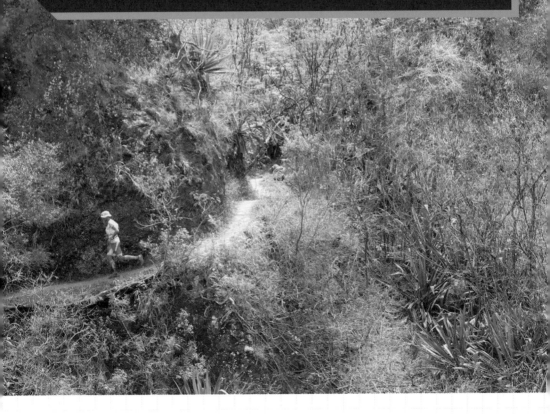

The science of ultra-marathon running is little different to the basic scientific principles of marathon running. Training is critical, with an emphasis on building up the length of the training to prepare the body both physiologically and psychologically for the challenge it will face. On race day, proper pacing is of course essential, running at a low exercise intensity to ensure that no lactic acid is produced, and the muscles are able to utilise fat stores and spare carbohydrate. Refuelling and rehydrating during an ultra are essential, and any runner who fails to do so will fail to finish. Some runners may factor in scheduled refuelling stops and even meals, during which their carbohydrate stores are replenished. As with marathons, practising refuelling while running in training is vital, so that the quantity and type of foods that can be eaten and tolerated is understood. The emphasis needs to be on carbohydrates, and carrying snacks and energy gels is a simple and effective way of maintaining energy levels. Continuous hydration is crucial, especially on warm days, and carrying water or isotonic drinks will ensure that sweating and heat loss can continue.

Psychologically, ultras present a much greater challenge than marathons, and using techniques such as 'zoning in', 'zoning out' and goal setting are vital. This may be more difficult to do in longer events because runners often experience sleep deprivation, which can make mental concentration and focus harder, and disrupt the body's circadian rhythms. Deciding whether to continue without sleep or to schedule short sleep breaks is a challenge that a number of ultra-runners face.

Many ultras will specify the clothing that runners need to carry with them, since the duration of the event means that climate variability is highly likely. Staying warm and dry when conditions are inclement is crucial for the safety and well-being of runners, and additional items not needed for marathon running could include a head torch, for night-time running, and a camel pack that holds fluid, for hydration.

Ultra-marathon running presents physical and mental challenges that exceed those experienced in marathon running, and it should not be attempted lightly. However, for many it provides a new and alternative challenge that explores the limits of human endurance.

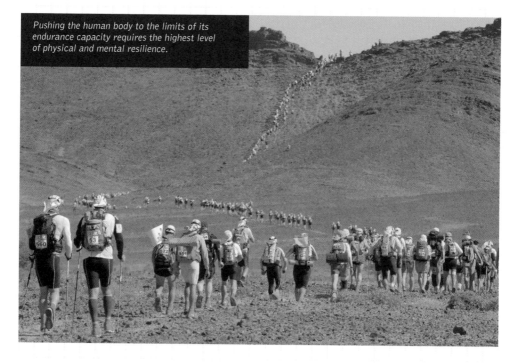

Pushing the human body to the limits of its endurance capacity requires the highest level of physical and mental resilience.

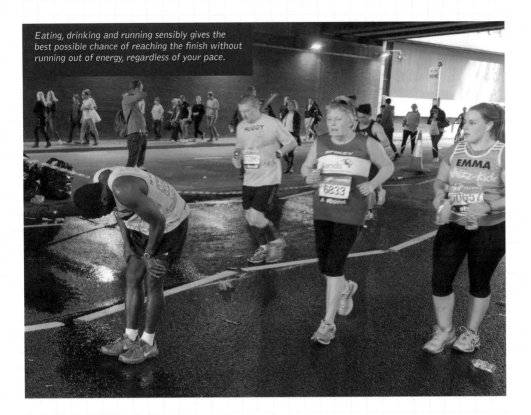

Eating, drinking and running sensibly gives the best possible chance of reaching the finish without running out of energy, regardless of your pace.

MYTH: *YOU'VE RUN OUT OF ENERGY WHEN YOU HIT THE WALL*

'I hit the wall.' Four words that strike fear into the heart of any marathon runner, and which almost certainly signify slow and painful progress over the last few miles of the race. 'The wall' has become synonymous with the point in a marathon – normally around 18–20 miles into the race – when everything comes to a grinding halt; an overwhelming feeling of fatigue combines with legs that feel heavy and unresponsive, and each stride requires significant effort. As a result, 'the wall' is commonly associated with running out of energy, with no more fuel left in the glycogen tank to sustain momentum to the finish line.

In fact, there is still plenty of energy left – but the body simply does not have the right type of fuel in the right place, so the trick is to work out how to use it.

The main muscles and muscle fibres that are employed when running will almost certainly have spent most if not all of their glycogen, but there should still be some reserves left in other muscles, and muscle fibres, that have done less work. A change in running style may help to unlock some of these reserves. Even if 'the wall' appears, there is also plenty of energy left from fat reserves. A 70kg (11st, or 154lb) runner with 15 per cent body fat will carry 10.5kg (23lb) of fat, which contains over 90,000 calories of energy – enough to sustain 30 marathons! However, fat is inefficient and cannot sustain fast running, so slowing down while still continuing to run will tap into these essential energy reserves, which are still in plentiful supply, even at the finish.

Training, planning, pacing and marginal gains can all contribute to a successful marathon experience.

RUN SMART RESOURCES

It is all too easy to overlook the basics, so this next section provides marathon runners of all standards with science-based, practical resources that can be used to support and fine-tune the successful completion of a marathon.

100 WAYS TO GO 1 PER CENT FASTER

While training is at the heart of marathon success, other lifestyle changes can enhance the way that you prepare your body to run 26.2 miles.

01 Follow a training programme that suits your needs.

02 Find a running partner to train with.

03 Consider joining a running club.

04 Build marathon training into your lifestyle.

05 Raise some sponsorship money – it helps with motivation.

06 Prioritise your weekly long run as a 'must do'.

07 Have a 'prehab' assessment to prevent injury.

08 Buy running shoes that suit your style.

09 Speak to a coach for personal-training advice.

10 Join an online forum for marathon runners to motivate and share experiences.

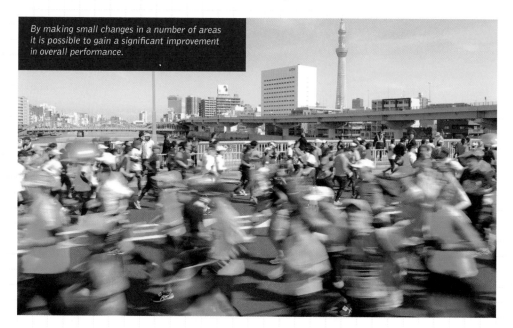

By making small changes in a number of areas it is possible to gain a significant improvement in overall performance.

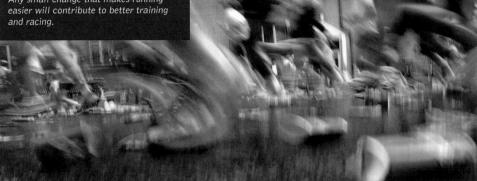

Any small change that makes running easier will contribute to better training and racing.

 11 Have a fitness assessment.

 12 Get your running style analysed.

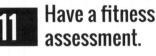 **13** Invest in a heart rate monitor.

14 Stretch regularly to avoid injury.

15 Progress your mileage steadily.

16 Fuel your training with plenty of carbohydrates.

 17 Rehydrate properly after training sessions.

 18 Reduce your alcohol intake.

 19 Losing 1kg (2.2lb) in weight reduces energy requirements by around 1 per cent.

 20 Choose different training routes to add variety to training.

21 Use warm-weather days for heat acclimation.

22 Warm up sensibly before training sessions.

23 Stretch regularly to increase your stride length.

24 Incorporate speed-endurance running into your training.

25 Use training to practise drinking while running.

26 Try race-day on-course drinks during training runs.

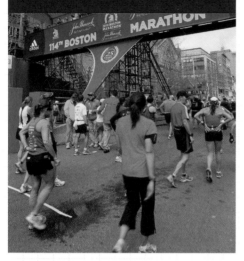

Marginal gains in performance benefit runners of all abilities, regardless of whether they start at the front or the back of the race.

27 Try race-day on-course gels during training runs.

28 Use hill running to develop leg strength.

29 Create your own microclimate with extra layers to prepare for hot conditions.

30 Train at the time you will be racing to set your body clock.

31 Incorporate races over shorter distances into your training.

32 Try out your race-day marathon kit in training.

33 Set a realistic target time for your marathon.

34 Work out your target race pace, and practise this in training.

35 Watch videos of previous marathons - seeing others finish should be a confidence boost.

36 Run with a GPS – although the race will have mile markers, knowing how far away the next one is can help.

37 Don't wear too many layers if conditions are wet.

38 As race day approaches, synchronise your bowel habits with an early start.

39 Take a daily multivitamin with iron as race day approaches.

40 Choose somewhere convenient to stay on the night before race day.

41 Familiarise yourself with the marathon route – where are the ups and downs?

42 Check out the race-day weather forecast.

43 Write out a check-list for everything you will need on race day.

44 Never run a marathon in new running shoes.

45 Plan your route to the start.

46 Keep eating plenty of carbohydrates as race day approaches.

47 Eat a banana – a large banana contains enough calories for 1 mile of running.

48 Do you really want to wear fancy dress? It will make the 26.2 miles much harder.

49 Stay off your feet as much as possible on the day before the race.

50 Don't eat anything unusual on the night before your marathon.

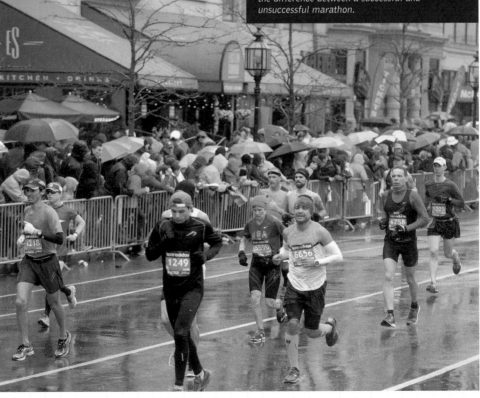

Being able to use the body's remaining energy reserves when the going gets tough can make the difference between a successful and unsuccessful marathon.

51 Choose a familiar, high-carbohydrate meal for 'marathon-eve'.

52 Stay hydrated over the days before the race.

 53 Check the colour of your urine to make sure it is a light straw colour.

54 Avoid alcohol on the day before your marathon.

55 Invest in some earplugs to aid a peaceful night's sleep.

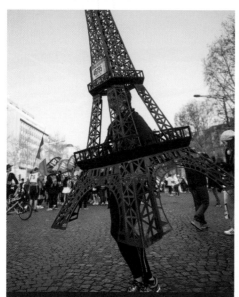

Wearing something that you feel comfortable in can make an important contribution to race day performance.

56 Male runners may find shaving hair from their chests aids sweating and helps them to keep cool on race day.

57 Trim your toenails or they may not last the distance.

 58 Keep a glass of water by your bedside on the night before the marathon.

 59 Wake with plenty of time for breakfast and to travel to the start.

 60 Set at least two alarm clocks.

61 Top-up fluid stores over breakfast.

62 Eat a familiar, light, carbohydrate breakfast.

63 A cup of coffee before the start will boost mental alertness.

64 Aim to rehydrate fully 1 hour before the start to reduce the need to pee when the race starts.

65 Take an isotonic drink or water bottle with you to the start.

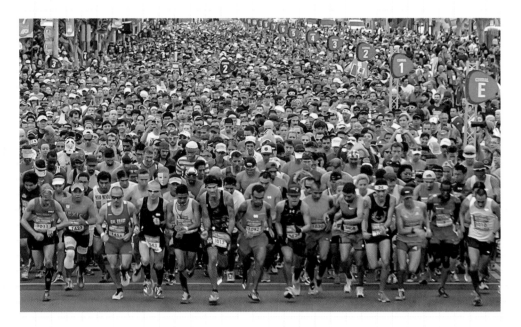

66 Arrive at the start with plenty of time for final preparations and going to the toilet.

67 Use petroleum jelly to lubricate all moving parts.

68 Use petroleum jelly on your feet to reduce the risk of blisters.

69 Tie your laces securely, but not so tightly that they restrict blood flow to the feet.

70 Check where the on-course toilets are so you know where you can have a quick pee-stop.

71 Don't wear extra layers even if it is cold at the start – it will warm up.

72 Run with an organised pacing group that matches your target time.

73 Choose a start pen containing runners of a similar pace.

74 Take time at the start to focus on your personal goals.

75 If you are a novice, remember the mantra 'complete not compete'.

76 Don't panic if you don't move when the start gun sounds.

77 Some races have a line marking the optimum route – follow it and you will avoid having to run extra distance.

78 Save as much energy as possible in the early stages – avoid chanting and high fiving.

79 On hot days, seek out the shade to stay cool.

80 On blustery days, use other runners as shields from the wind.

81 Make use of on-course drinks stations – taking frequent, small sips is better than gulping large volumes.

82 Use isotonic drinks to replace fluid, fuel and electrolytes.

83 On-course gels will replace glycogen and provide an energy boost.

84 Eat a jelly baby! Six will provide energy for around 1 mile of running.

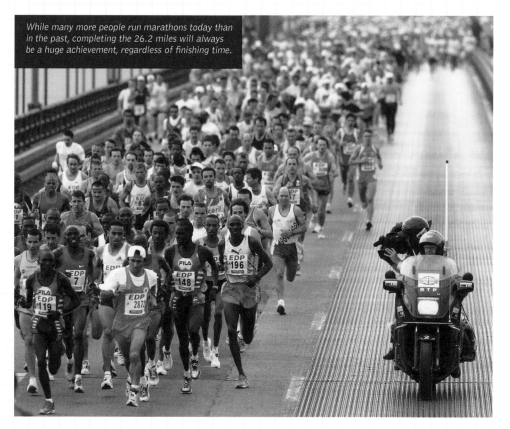

While many more people run marathons today than in the past, completing the 26.2 miles will always be a huge achievement, regardless of finishing time.

85 If you carry a phone, arrange for friends to make motivational calls at regular intervals.

86 If there are showers on course, use them to cool down.

87 Reset the distance – as the race unfolds you no longer have 26.2 miles left to complete.

88 Scientists have shown that listening to music can motivate runners.

89 Don't slump forwards as you tire. Run tall – it is easier on the lungs, and faster.

90 In major marathons, use the crowd's cheering to motivate you to finish.

91 Zone in, to focus on your own body and your running pace.

92 Zone out, to let the crowd and atmosphere carry you towards the finish line.

93 Have friends and family on course to give you encouragement.

94 To cope with mental fatigue recite a mantra such as "I will I can" or even sing a song in your head.

95 Count your strides, and when you reach a number such as 100, start again.

96 Visualise crossing the finish line, and the euphoria that you will feel.

97 When the going gets tough, plod or walk. Don't stop.

98 Taste something sweet. Scientists have found that this can give a short-term mental and physical boost.

99 Try changing your stride length to use different muscle fibres and energy reserves.

100 No matter how tired you are, summon your last reserves of energy to run tall and strong and look good as you approach and cross the finish line.

BASIC TRAINING PROGRAMME

The basic training programme is designed for those who have busy lifestyles, and for whom marathon running is something new.

This is a training plan for runners who may well be first-timers, and whose aim is to complete the distance, not to race 26.2 miles and achieve a personal-best time. Crucial to the programme is the use of higher-intensity interval and fartlek running to gain maximum returns from the time invested in training. The programme includes a weekly extension of the 'long run', which progresses in a way that builds cardiovascular and local muscular endurance, while minimising the risk of injury.

KEY	CP = conversational pace TDP = tolerable discomfort pace

WEEK 1
Day 1: 20-minute steady run at conversation pace (CP).
Day 2: 30-minute steady run at CP.
Day 3: Long run – 5 miles at slow, comfortable pace.

WEEK 2
Day 1: 30-minute steady run at CP.
Day 2: 30-minute steady run at CP.
Day 3: Long run – 6 miles at slow, comfortable pace.

WEEK 3
Day 1: 40-minute steady run at CP.
Day 2: 30-minute steady run at CP.
Day 3: Long run – 7 miles at slow, comfortable pace.

WEEK 4
Day 1: 20-minute tempo run at tolerable discomfort pace (TDP).
Day 2: 35-minute steady run at CP.
Day 3: Long run – 8 miles at slow, comfortable pace.

WEEK 5
Day 1: 30-minute tempo run at TDP.
Day 2: 40-minute steady run at CP.
Day 3: Long run – 9 miles at slow, comfortable pace.

WEEK 6
Day 1: 30-minute steady run that includes eight 60-second fast bursts with 2 minutes' jog recovery after each burst.
Day 2: 30-minute steady run at CP.
Day 3: 40-minute steady run at CP.
Day 4: Long run – 10 miles at slow, comfortable pace.

WEEK 7
Day 1: 40-minute steady run at CP.
Day 2: 30-minute tempo run at TDP.
Day 3: 20-minute recovery run at slow pace.
Day 4: Long run – 11 miles at slow, comfortable pace.

WEEK 8
Day 1: 40-minute steady run that includes ten 60-second fast bursts with 2 minutes' jog recovery after each burst.
Day 2: 30-minute steady run at CP.
Day 3: 25-minute run at TDP.
Day 4: Long run – 12 miles at slow, comfortable pace.

WEEK 9
Day 1: 30-minute steady run at CP.
Day 2: 50-minute steady run that includes ten 60-second fast bursts with 2 minutes' jog recovery after each burst.
Day 3: 30-minute tempo run at TDP.
Day 4: Long run – 13 miles at slow, comfortable pace.

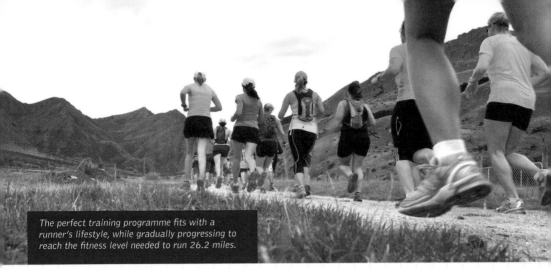

The perfect training programme fits with a runner's lifestyle, while gradually progressing to reach the fitness level needed to run 26.2 miles.

WEEK 10
Day 1: 40-minute steady run at CP.
Day 2: 30-minute steady run at CP.
Day 3: 40-minute fartlek session – aim for six fast bursts of varying length.
Day 4: Long run – 14 miles at slow, comfortable pace.

WEEK 11
Day 1: 40-minute steady run at CP.
Day 2: 30-minute tempo run at TDP.
Day 3: 40-minute fartlek session – aim for eight fast bursts of varying length.
Day 4: Long run – 15 miles at slow, comfortable pace.

WEEK 12
Day 1: 40-minute steady run at CP.
Day 2: 60-minute steady run at CP.
Day 3: 50-minute steady run that includes ten 60-second fast bursts with 2 minutes' jog recovery after each burst.
Day 4: Long run – 16 miles at slow, comfortable pace.

WEEK 13
Day 1: 40-minute steady run at CP.
Day 2: 60-minute steady run at CP.
Day 3: 50-minute fartlek run that includes ten fast bursts of varying duration.
Day 4: Long run – 18 miles at slow, comfortable pace.

WEEK 14
Day 1: 30-minute steady run at CP.
Day 2: 45-minute steady run at CP.
Day 3: Long run – 20–22 miles at slow, comfortable pace.

WEEK 15
Day 1: 20-minute steady run at CP.
Day 2: 30-minute steady run at CP.
Day 3: Long run – 12–13 miles at slow, comfortable pace.

WEEK 16
Day 1: 20-minute steady run at CP.
Day 2: 30-minute steady run at CP.
Day 3: Long run – 8 miles at slow, comfortable pace.

WEEK 17
Marathon

ADVANCED TRAINING PROGRAMME

The advanced training programme is designed for runners who may be more experienced, and who are prepared to devote significant time and energy to their marathon training.

This programme involves more training days and a higher weekly mileage than the basic training programme, but the fundamental principles remain the same – a gradual increase in the weekly long run, and the incorporation of higher-intensity training to develop cardiovascular fitness and leg strength. With a programme of this nature, recovery time is critical, even for experienced runners, providing the all-important opportunity for muscle repair and physiological adaptations to the stimulus of training to occur.

KEY	CP = conversational pace TDP = tolerable discomfort pace

WEEK 1
Day 1: 20-minute steady run at conversation pace CP.
Day 2: 30-minute steady run at CP.
Day 3: Hill session – four 1-minute uphill runs, jogging back down to recover. Take 5 minutes' rest, then repeat.
Day 4: Long run – 6 miles at slow, comfortable pace.

WEEK 2
Day 1: 30-minute steady run at CP.
Day 2: 25-minute fartlek session including five bursts of faster running.
Day 3: 40-minute steady run at CP.
Day 4: Long run – 7 miles at slow, comfortable pace.

WEEK 3
Day 1: 40-minute steady run at CP.
Day 2: 40-minute steady run at CP.
Day 3: 20-minute fast tempo run at tolerable discomfort pace (TDP).
Day 4: Long run – 8 miles at slow, comfortable pace.

WEEK 4
Day 1: 30-minute tempo run.
Day 2: 40-minute steady run at CP.
Day 3: 30-minute fartlek session including six faster bursts.
Day 4: Long run – 9 miles at slow, comfortable pace.

WEEK 5
Day 1: 30-minute tempo run at TDP.
Day 2: 40-minute steady run at CP.
Day 3: Hill session: four 2-minute uphill runs, jog to bottom to recover. Take 5 minutes' rest, then repeat twice.
Day 4: 20-minute steady run at CP.
Day 5: Long run – 10 miles at slow, comfortable pace.

WEEK 6
Day 1: 40-minute steady run that includes ten 60-second fast bursts with 2 minutes' jog recovery after each burst.
Day 2: 40-minute steady run at CP.

Day 3: Hill session: four 2-minute uphill runs, jog to bottom to recover. Take 5 minutes' rest, then repeat twice.
Day 4: 40-minute steady run at CP.
Day 5: Long run – 12 miles at slow, comfortable pace.

WEEK 7
Day 1: 40-minute steady run at CP.
Day 2: Hill session: four 2-minute uphill runs, jog to bottom to recover. Take 5 minutes' rest, then repeat twice.
Day 3: 30-minute tempo run at TDP.
Day 4: 40-minute fartlek session with eight faster bursts.
Day 5: Long run – 13 miles at steady pace (or a half-marathon race).

WEEK 8
Day 1: 40-minute steady run that includes ten 60-second fast bursts with 2 minutes' jog recovery after each burst.
Day 2: 50-minute steady run at CP.
Day 3: Hill session: four 2 minute uphill runs, jog to bottom to recover. Take 5 minutes' rest, then repeat twice.
Day 4: 30-minute run at TDP.
Day 5: Long run – 14 miles at slow, comfortable pace.

WEEK 9
Day 1: 50-minute steady run at CP.
Day 2: 50-minute steady run that includes ten 2-minute faster bursts with 2 minutes' jog recovery after each burst.
Day 3: 30-minute tempo run at TDP.
Day 4: 50-minute fartlek session.
Day 5: Long run – 16 miles at slow, comfortable pace.

WEEK 10
Day 1: 60-minute steady run at CP.
Day 2: 40-minute fartlek session.
Day 3: 60-minute steady run at CP.
Day 4: 30-minute tempo session at TDP.
Day 5: Long run – 18 miles at slow, comfortable pace.

WEEK 11
Day 1: 60-minute steady run at CP.
Day 2: 40-minute fartlek session.
Day 3: 60-minute steady run at CP.
Day 4: Hill session: four 2 minute uphill runs, jog to bottom to recover. Take 5 minutes' rest, then repeat twice.
Day 5: Long run – 19 miles at slow, comfortable pace.

WEEK 12
Day 1: 60-minute steady run at CP.
Day 2: 40-minute fartlek session.
Day 3: 60-minute steady run at CP.
Day 4: 50-minute steady run that includes eight 2-minute fast bursts with 3 minutes' jog recovery after each burst.
Day 5: Long run – 20 miles at slow, comfortable pace.

WEEK 13
Day 1: 40-minute steady run at CP.
Day 2: 60-minute steady run at CP.
Day 3: 50-minute fartlek run that includes 10 faster bursts of varying duration.
Day 4: Long run – 20–22 miles at slow, comfortable pace.

WEEK 14
Day 1: 30-minute steady run at CP.
Day 2: 60-minute steady run at CP.
Day 3: 60-minute steady run at CP.
Day 4: Long run – 20–23 miles at slow, comfortable pace.

WEEK 15
Day 1: 20-minute steady run at CP.
Day 2: 30-minute steady run at CP.
Day 3: Long run – 12–13 miles at slow, comfortable pace.

WEEK 16
Day 1: 20-minute steady run at CP.
Day 2: 30-minute steady run at CP.
Day 3: Long run – 8 miles at slow, comfortable pace.

WEEK 17
Marathon

TRAINING CALENDAR

This visual guide to the training programmes outlined on pages 176–179 shows at a glance what you should be doing from week to week.

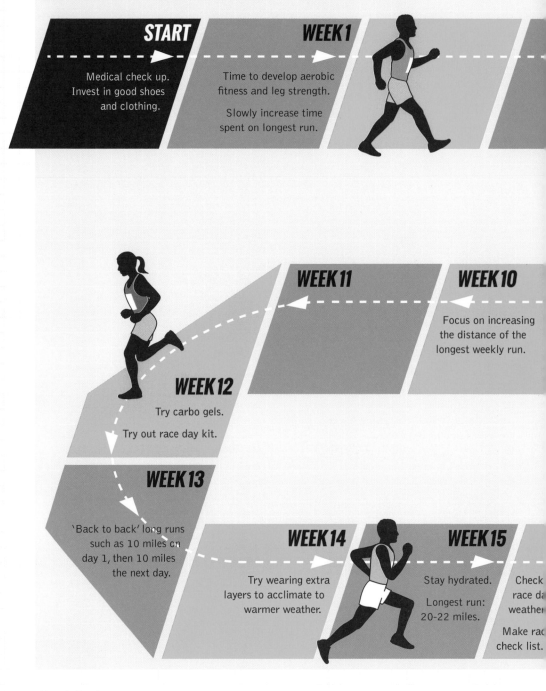

START
Medical check up. Invest in good shoes and clothing.

WEEK 1
Time to develop aerobic fitness and leg strength.

Slowly increase time spent on longest run.

WEEK 11

WEEK 10
Focus on increasing the distance of the longest weekly run.

WEEK 12
Try carbo gels.

Try out race day kit.

WEEK 13
'Back to back' long runs such as 10 miles on day 1, then 10 miles the next day.

WEEK 14
Try wearing extra layers to acclimate to warmer weather.

WEEK 15
Stay hydrated.

Longest run: 20-22 miles.

Check race da weather

Make rac check list.

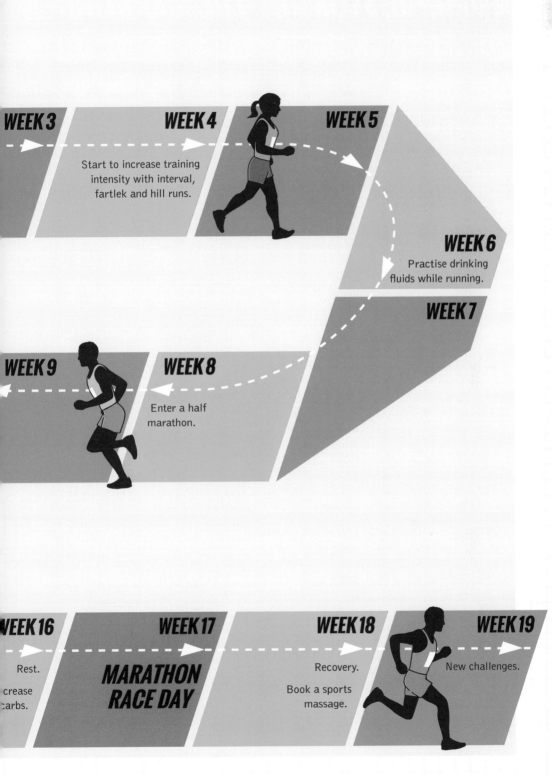

WEEK 3

WEEK 4
Start to increase training intensity with interval, fartlek and hill runs.

WEEK 5

WEEK 6
Practise drinking fluids while running.

WEEK 7

WEEK 8
Enter a half marathon.

WEEK 9

WEEK 16
Rest.
crease
arbs.

WEEK 17
MARATHON RACE DAY

WEEK 18
Recovery.
Book a sports massage.

WEEK 19
New challenges.

A BRIEF HISTORY OF THE MARATHON

From Ancient Greece to the Modern Olympics, and in towns and cities around the world, marathons have become a pinnacle of achievement for many endurance runners.

Legend tells us that the marathon originates from a day in around 490 BC, when the Greek messenger Pheidippides ran from the battlefields of Marathon near Sparta to Athens in order to pronounce victory for the Greeks over their warring rivals, the Persians. On uttering the words 'we have won', unfortunately Pheidippides promptly dropped dead. Although the exact cause of his demise will always remain a mystery, it may well have been due to a combination of heat exhaustion and dehydration, both of which have been explored in this book. As with many legends of this nature, there are conflicting views about its accuracy. Moreover, the fact that there were two distinct routes from Sparta to Athens, both of differing distances, makes it hard to know exactly how far Pheidippides had run.

It is also a legend that would have remained largely unheard of had it not been for the French Baron, Pierre de Coubertin, who had the inspiration to launch the modern Olympic Games in Athens in 1896, based on the Olympic competitions previously held in Ancient Greece. De Coubertin and his colleagues wanted an event to be included that would be a focal point of the Games, celebrating the ancient glory of Greece. Replicating Pheidippides' epic run was deemed to be the answer. The first Olympic Champion was, appropriately, the Greek runner Spyridon Louis, who completed the race in a time of just under three hours, although in the early years of marathon running the distance was not fixed and tended to be approximately 25 miles. For the London Olympic Games in 1908, the race started at the Royal Family's Windsor Castle, before finishing 26 miles away at The Great Stadium in White City, West London. In order that the runners finished the race in front of the Royal Box, they had to complete a further partial lap of the stadium's track that totalled 385 yards.

The marathon distance continued to vary until, in 1921, the International Amateur Athletics Federations decreed that the official distance for the marathon should be the 26 miles 385 yards (42.195 kilometres) used for the 1908 London Olympics, and it is a distance that remains in place today.

For many years to come, marathon running remained the domain of hardened, dedicated male runners. Indeed, the first female Olympic marathon was not held until the 1984 Olympic Games in Los Angeles. However, during the 1970s and 1980s, things started to change, and marathon running began to grow in popularity and increasingly became mass-participation events. The American athlete Frank Shorter became a national hero when he became Olympic Marathon Champion in 1972, and this victory sparked a surge of enthusiasm for running, and marathons in particular. Major cities such as New York, Boston and Chicago saw entry fields for their marathons start to grow rapidly, and as other cities around the world launched their own annual marathon, the global growth in popularity of this type of running began. When the London Marathon was launched in 1981, one of its co-founders, Chris Brasher, described the marathon as 'suburban man's Everest', and in many ways this comment sums up what marathons are, and have become. Running a marathon is an immense challenge, and completing one is an accomplishment that any runner should be rightly proud of. However, today, running 26.2 miles is something that almost anyone, regardless of age or ability, can achieve, provided they have the right dedication, preparation and training. You do not need to be a serious runner who dedicates his or her life to running in order to complete the distance, and with the right use of correct advice and science, finishing a marathon really is possible for many, not just a few.

The organisers of today's marathons have a very different mindset from those who arranged the races of 50 or more years ago – today they expect many runners to run slowly, they know that some will need to walk part of the distance, and they don't expect everyone to have finished within 4 hours. Marathons are planned to support those who take far longer, and for whom the aim is – first and foremost – to complete the distance, often for the one and only time in their lives.

Had sports science been available to support long-distance running in 490 BC, it is quite possible that Pheidippides would not have died when he reached Athens. Unfortunately for him it was not, and in fact very little was understood about the science of endurance running for many years to come. When the US runner Thomas Hicks won the 1904 Olympic marathon in St Louis, his support team barred him from taking water, and instead gave him copious quantities of alcohol and egg whites, with further 'help' from the now-banned stimulant strychnine. Not much is known about training schedules in that era,

although ultra-endurance events involving epic foot races over many sleep-deprived days were commonplace.

In the early 20th century, two global challenges had an impact on the application of scientific knowledge to human performance. The first of these was the exploration of the world's polar regions, and the consequent desire to better understand the specific nutritional needs of those embarking on long journeys to remote areas. The second challenge was the quest to conquer the world's highest mountains, and of course the race to be the first to climb Mount Everest in the Himalayas. One of the first scientists to leave the laboratory behind and accompany mountaineering expeditions to take measurements on humans in the oxygen-deprived atmosphere of the high mountains was British physiologist and mountaineer Griffith Pugh. Pugh's research marked the start of a much greater comprehension of how extreme exercise affects the human body, and today the application of science to endurance performance has evolved in the same way, and over the same time period, that marathon running has grown in popularity.

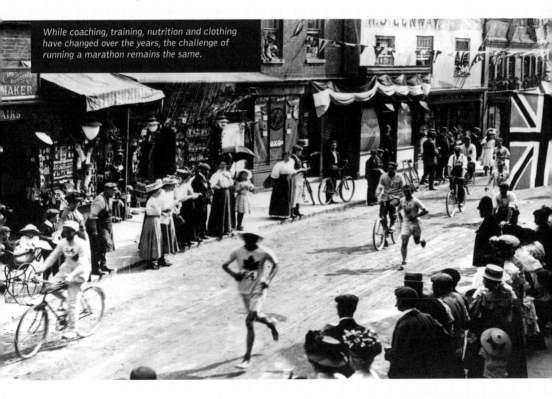

While coaching, training, nutrition and clothing have changed over the years, the challenge of running a marathon remains the same.

SOME USEFUL TABLES

Throughout this book we have measured distances in miles, since that is how marathons are frequently measured, but of course you may prefer to train and run using kilometres as your guide instead. There are many online convertors, and running aids usually offer the option of measuring distance in either miles or kilometres, but for ease of reference, here are the figures.

MILES TO KILOMETRES CONVERSION TABLE

Miles	Kilometres	Miles	kilometres
1	1.6	14	22.5
2	3.2	15	24
3	4.8	16	25.7
4	6.4	17	27.4
5	8	18	29
6	9.7	19	30.6
7	11.3	20	32.2
8	12.9	21	33.8
9	14.5	22	35.4
10	16.1	23	37
11	17.7	24	38.6
12	19.3	25	40.2
13	20.9	26.2	42.2

RUNNING PACE TABLE IN MILES AND KILOMETRES

Mile/h	Km/h	Min/mile	Min/km	400m	5k	10k	½ mara	Mara
4.00	6.44	15.00	9.19	3.44	46.35	1.33.10	3.16.38	6.33.17
4.20	6.76	14.17	8.53	3.33	44.25	1.28.50	3.07.15	6.14.29
4.35	7.00	13.48	8.34	3.26	42.50	1.25.40	3.00.55	6.01.49
4.40	7.08	13.38	8.28	3.23	42.20	1.24.40	2.58.43	5.57.27
4.60	7.40	13.03	8.06	3.14	40.30	1.21.00	2.51.05	5.42.09
4.80	7.72	12.30	7.46	3.06	38.50	1.17.40	2.43.52	5.27.44
4.97	8.00	12.04	7.30	3.00	37.30	1.15.00	2.38.11	5.16.22
5.00	8.05	12.00	7.27	2.59	37.15	1.14.30	2.37.19	5.14.38
5.20	8.37	11.32	7.10	2.52	35.50	1.11.40	2.31.12	5.02.23
5.40	8.69	11.07	6.54	2.46	34.30	1.09.00	2.25.44	4.51.28
5.59	9.00	10.44	6.40	2.40	33.20	1.06.40	2.20.42	4.41.25
5.60	9.01	10.43	6.39	2.40	33.15	1.06.30	2.20.29	4.40.59
5.80	9.33	10.21	6.26	2.34	32.10	1.04.20	2.15.41	4.31.22
6.00	9.66	10.00	6.13	2.29	31.05	1.02.10	2.11.06	4.22.11
6.20	9.98	9.41	6.01	2.24	30.05	1.00.10	2.06.57	4.13.53
6.21	10.00	9.39	6.00	2.24	30.00	1.00.00	2.06.30	4.13.01
6.40	10.30	9.23	5.50	2.20	29.10	0.58.20	2.03.01	4.06.01
6.60	10.62	9.05	5.39	2.16	28.15	0.56.30	1.59.05	3.58.09
6.80	10.94	8.49	5.29	2.12	27.25	0.54.50	1.55.35	3.51.10
6.84	11.00	8.47	5.27	2.11	27.15	0.54.30	1.55.09	3.50.17

Mile/h	Km/h	Min/mile	Min/km	400m	5k	10k	½ mara	Mara
7.00	11.27	8.34	5.20	2.08	26.40	0.53.20	1.52.18	3.44.36
7.20	11.59	8.20	5.11	2.04	25.55	0.51.50	1.49.15	3.38.29
7.40	11.91	8.06	5.02	2.01	25.10	0.50.20	1.46.11	3.32.22
7.46	12.00	8.03	5.00	2.00	25.00	0.50.00	1.45.32	3.31.04
7.60	12.23	7.54	4.54	1.58	24.30	0.49.00	1.43.34	3.27.08
7.80	12.55	7.42	4.47	1.55	23.55	0.47.50	1.40.57	3.21.53
8.00	12.87	7.30	4.40	1.52	23.20	0.46.40	1.38.19	3.16.38
8.08	13.00	7.26	4.37	1.51	23.05	0.46.10	1.37.27	3.14.54
8.20	13.20	7.19	4.33	1.49	22.45	0.45.55	1.35.55	3.11.50
8.40	13.52	7.09	4.26	1.46	22.10	0.44.20	1.33.44	3.07.28
8.60	13.84	6.59	4.20	1.44	21.40	0.43.20	1.31.33	3.03.06
8.70	14.00	6.54	4.17	1.43	21.25	0.42.50	1.30.27	3.00.55
8.80	14.16	6.49	4.14	1.42	21.10	0.42.20	1.29.22	2.58.43
9.00	14.48	6.40	4.09	1.40	20.45	0.41.30	1.27.24	2.54.48
9.20	14.81	6.31	4.03	1.37	20.15	0.40.30	1.25.26	2.50.52
9.32	15.00	6.26	4.00	1.36	20.00	0.40.00	1.24.20	2.48.40
9.40	15.13	6.23	3.58	1.35	19.50	0.39.40	1.23.41	2.47.22
9.60	15.45	6.15	3.53	1.33	19.25	0.38.50	1.21.56	2.43.52
9.80	15.77	6.07	3.48	1.31	19.00	0.38.00	1.20.11	2.40.22
9.94	16.00	6.02	3.45	1.30	18.45	0.37.30	1.19.06	2.38.11
10.00	16.09	6.00	3.44	1.30	18.40	0.37.20	1.18.39	2.37.19
10.20	16.42	5.53	3.39	1.28	18.15	0.36.30	1.17.08	2.34.15
10.40	16.74	5.46	3.35	1.26	17.55	0.35.50	1.15.36	2.31.12
10.56	17.00	5.41	3.32	1.25	17.40	0.35.20	1.14.30	2.29.01
10.60	17.06	5.40	3.31	1.24	17.35	0.35.10	1.14.17	2.28.34
10.80	17.38	5.33	3.27	1.23	17.15	0.34.30	1.12.45	2.25.31
11.00	17.70	5.27	3.23	1.21	16.55	0.33.50	1.11.27	2.22.54
11.18	18.00	5.22	3.20	1.20	16.40	0.33.20	1.10.21	2.20.42
11.20	18.02	5.21	3.20	1.20	16.40	0.33.20	1.10.08	2.20.16
11.40	18.35	5.16	3.16	1.18	16.20	0.32.40	1.09.03	2.18.05
11.60	18.67	5.10	3.13	1.17	16.05	0.32.10	1.07.44	2.15.28
11.80	18.99	5.05	3.10	1.16	15.50	0.31.40	1.06.38	2.13.17
11.81	19.00	5.05	3.09	1.16	15.45	0.31.30	1.06.38	2.13.17
12.00	19.31	5.00	3.06	1.14	15.30	0.31.00	1.05.33	2.11.06
12.20	19.63	4.55	3.03	1.13	15.15	0.30.30	1.04.27	2.08.55
12.40	19.96	4.50	3.00	1.12	15.00	0.30.00	1.03.22	2.06.43
12.43	20.00	4.50	3.00	1.12	15.00	0.30.00	1.03.22	2.06.43
12.60	20.28	4.46	2.58	1.11	14.50	0.29.40	1.02.29	2.04.59
12.80	20.60	4.41	2.55	1.10	14.35	0.29.10	1.01.24	2.02.47
13.00	20.92	4.37	2.52	1.09	14.20	0.28.40	1.00.31	2.01.03

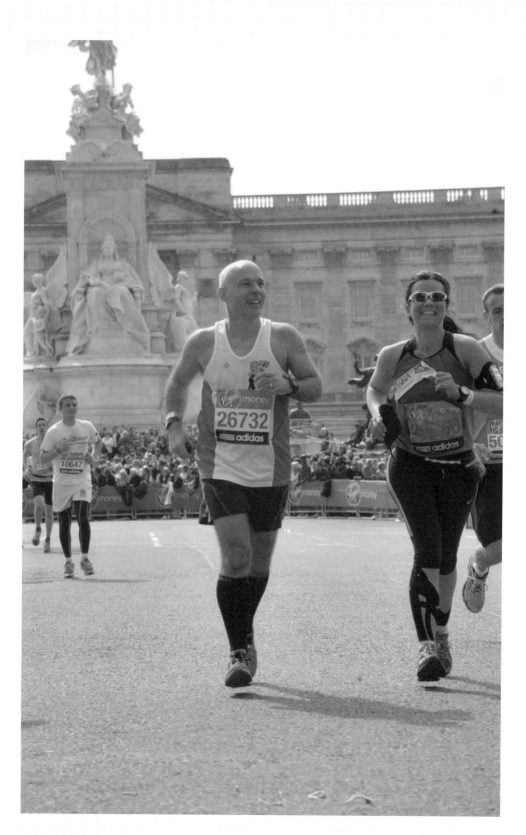

ABOUT THE AUTHOR

John Brewer is Professor of Applied Sports Science at St Mary's University, Twickenham. He is one of the UK's leading sports scientists and marathon specialists, due to his extensive research background in marathon running and his experience as a marathon runner. He is an advisor to the London Marathon, as well as a 19-time runner of the event. He is also a London Marathon celebrity chaperone, assisting media personalities in completing the course. He is a regular contributor to various running magazines and is a popular media commentator on sports science having worked with a number of major sports organisations and teams, including the Football Association, England Football team, Team GB Handball team and England Cricket team. John Brewer is the author of the official *London 2012 Olympic Games Track Athletics Training Guide.*

INDEX

A

acclimation 106
aches and pains 17, 73,
    105, 120, 145–6
adenosine triphosphate
    (ATP) 16, 22
adrenalin 16, 28
age 50–1
ageing 51, 53
alcohol 125, 132–3
altitude, running at 70–1
appetite loss 119
'association' technique 34

B

bag, kit 132, 151
Berlin Marathon,
    Germany 159
biomechanics 27, 42–3,
    48–9, 68
blisters 33, 49, 107, 145–6,
    152
blood flow/supply 14, 17,
    22, 23, 24, 32, 33, 49,
    75, 104
blood pressure 53
bloodstream 24, 32, 33,
    66
body clock 76–7
body temperature see core
    temperature
bodyweight and size 15, 20,
    37, 39, 44, 47, 56, 72, 86,
    95, 107
Boston Marathon, USA
    158–9
brains 32, 75
Brasher, Chris 182
breakfast, race-day 133,
    136–7
breathing 16, 24, 25, 66–7,
    145, 146

C

caffeine 138
calories burnt 15, 17, 36, 53,
    73, 95, 101, 125, 147
carbo gels see gels, energy
carbohydrates 12, 15, 16, 17,
    30, 36, 37, 38–9, 55, 72, 73,
    100–1, 103, 111–12, 124,
    125, 129, 136, 142, 152
cardiovascular system
    see heart; lungs; oxygen
    transportation
chafing 49, 107, 123, 133,
    145, 152
Chicago Marathon, USA
    159
circadian rhythms 40, 76–7
clothing 13, 25, 48–9, 80,
    106–7, 123, 129, 130–1
coaches, personal 91
coconut water 103
Coe, Sebastian 20
colds and coughs 116–17
collapsing 75
compression socks 49
core/body temperature
    12, 13, 14, 16, 17, 22, 25,
    38, 56, 65, 74–5, 77,
    104, 151
cramp 17, 163
cross-training 108–9
cycling 108, 157
cytokines 40–1

D

Death Valley Marathon,
    USA 160
dehydration 17, 33, 38–9, 67,
    72–3, 75, 95, 102–3, 133,
    138–9, 146
delayed onset muscle
    soreness (DOMS) 152
diet see nutrition

'dissociation' technique 34–5
drinks 13, 33, 38–9, 65,
    72–3, 75, 102–3, 123,
    138–9, 146, 152
drive phase 27
duathlons 156–7
dynamic stretches 104

E

electrolytes 17, 38–9, 73,
    103, 139, 152, 163
endorphins 17, 118
energy drinks 39, 73
    see also gels, energy;
        isotonic/sports drinks
energy expenditure 15, 17,
    36–7, 73
energy production 16, 17,
    20, 22, 24–5, 60
energy storage see
    carbohydrates; fat stores;
    liver
erythropoietin 71
Everest Marathon,
    Nepal 160

F

fartlek running 98
fast twitch muscles 60
fat diets 100, 136
fat stores 15, 16, 17, 21, 30,
    37, 55, 65, 95, 125, 165
fatigue 16, 17, 26, 62, 72, 75,
    95, 119, 135, 145, 146
fitness, assessing your 86–7
fitness regression 58
fluid loss 17, 33, 38–9, 72–3,
    75, 95, 102–3, 138–9
food see nutrition
foot strikes 42–3
footwear 13, 48–9, 87, 111
friends/running clubs 80, 83,
    90, 91

G

gait cycles 27
Gatorade 39
gels, energy 33, 123, 137, 139, 142
gender 54–6
genetics 54, 55, 56
glucose 32
glycogen 15, 16, 17, 30, 32, 36, 37, 40, 44, 65, 72, 73, 89, 124, 125, 137, 146, 165
glycogen synthase 37, 73, 101
goal setting 114–15, 153, 156–7
GPS 68
guts 33

H

haemoglobin 22, 24, 54, 66, 70–1, 101
half-marathons 115, 156
heart rate 16, 17, 22, 23, 24–5, 32, 65, 68, 86, 104, 120
heart rate monitors 68, 99, 113
hearts 32, 54, 66, 75, 108
heat loss 14, 17, 25, 49
Hicks, Thomas 38, 183
high intensity training 18, 98–9
history of marathons 182–3
hydration 12, 38–9, 72–3, 75, 95, 102–3, 124, 129, 133, 138–9, 146, 152
hyperthermia 38, 75, 130
hyponatremia 139

I

ice baths 152
illness 13, 53, 85, 95, 116–17, 120

immune system 40
impact forces 26–7, 33, 49, 108
improvements, making 58–9
injury risk and prevention 13, 49, 62, 83, 85, 87, 95, 104, 108, 109, 110–12, 119, 150
interval training 59, 62, 98–9
iron supplements 101
isotonic/sports drinks 39, 73, 102, 103, 123, 138–9, 152, 163

J

jet lag 77

K

kidneys 32–3
Krebs cycle 16

L

laboratory assessments, sports science 86–7
lactic acid 17, 23, 49, 59, 62, 72, 86, 99, 104–5, 121
layers, clothing 106–7, 130–1
ligaments see muscles, ligaments and tendons
light-headedness 32
liver 32, 36, 40
London Marathon, UK 18, 102, 159
longevity 53
low intensity training 18, 98–9
lungs 32, 54, 66–7, 70, 108, 117, 146

M

marathons
   100 ways to go faster 168–75
   abroad 156
   are they bad for you? 111
   history of 182–3
   hitting the wall 165
   how many can be run in a year? 121
   last few hours before start 132–3
   the Majors 158–9
   making it through tough times 64–5
   marginal gains 59
   mass-participation starts 140–1, 143
   metabolic demands 14–15
   post-marathon disappointment 150
   post-marathon running 153
   race-day psychology 134–5
   time of day 76–7
   walking impact on time 147
   what happens to your body during 16–17
   your vital organs 32–3
marginal gains 59
massage 152
medical advice 110–11, 112, 117
Medoc Marathon, France 161
meeting points 129, 151
mental preparation 12–13, 22, 34–5, 45, 132
metabolic demands 14–15
miles to kilometre conversion tables 185–6
milk-based drinks 103

mitochondria 16
mood changes 120
muscle loss 51
muscles, ligaments and
    tendons 12, 14, 16, 17,
    20, 22, 23, 24, 32, 37, 40,
    49, 54, 60, 62, 66, 70, 73,
    104, 121, 124, 146, 152,
    163, 165
music 83
myths, marathon 18, 31,
    45, 53, 55, 57, 61, 62, 83,
    85, 95, 111, 121

N

nasal strips 67, 145
'negative split' strategy
    44
nerves, race-day 134–5
New York Marathon, USA
    158, 159
North Dorset Villages
    Marathon, UK 161
North Pole Marathon,
    North Pole 160–1
number allocation 128
nutrition 12, 13, 33, 36–7,
    50, 65, 100–1, 111–12,
    124, 125, 129, 132, 133,
    136–7, 142, 152

O

older runners 50–1
orthotics 49
overheating 74–5, 130
overtaking and being
    overtaken 31
overtraining 118–20
oxygen transportation 12,
    22, 32, 54, 66, 70, 108
oxygen uptake 16, 17, 20–1,
    24–5, 30, 50, 51, 54, 62, 65,
    66, 75, 86, 99, 104

P

pace chart 92
pacers 46
pacing 13, 28–30, 31, 44, 59,
    65, 144–5
petroleum jelly 133
Pheidippides 37, 53, 182
physiotherapists 110–11, 112
positivity 17, 135, 145
potassium 17, 39
pre-marathon races 115
pre-race plans 128–9
prehab 110–11
pronation 49
protein 37, 40, 100, 103,
    136
psychology, marathon 17,
    34–5, 45, 65, 134–5, 142,
    143, 145
    see also mental
    preparation
Pugh, Griffiths 70, 183

R

race-day
    coping with 140–1
    getting a good start
        140–1, 143
    hydration 138–9
    last few hours 132–3
    nutrition 136–7, 143
    psychology 134–5, 142,
        143, 145, 146
    strategy 144–6
races, shorter 115, 156–7
Radcliffe, Paula 42, 54–5
recovery 13, 37, 59, 61,
    72–3, 83, 103, 104–5, 119,
    120, 150–3
regression, fitness 58
relative exercise intensity
    (REI) 21
relaxation 17, 145

respiratory system 66–7
Riegel, Pete 115
risk of injury/illness 13
route, know the route 140
routes, varying running 83
running intensity/speed
    20–1, 28–30, 44–5, 59, 62,
    86–7, 98, 114, 147
running kit 48–9, 80
running, post-marathon
    153
running style 42–3, 53,
    86–7, 146

S

salt tablets 163
sarcopenia 51
shoes, running 13, 48–9,
    87, 111
Shorter, Frank 182
shorts 49
skin 33, 74–5
sleep 40–1, 112, 119, 133
slow twitch muscles 60
snacks 133, 137
socks 49
sodium 17, 39, 163
space blankets 151
spectators 137, 141, 145
speed-endurance training
    60, 62
sports bras 49
sports drinks see isotonic/
    sports drinks
sports science overview
    12–13
start times, marathon
    76–7
static stretching 104
stitch 146
stomach 33, 146
strategies and tactics,
    race 44, 46, 59
stresses on the body 13

stretches 104, 105, 152
strides 26–7, 42–3, 47
sun cream 131
supplements, food 101
sweating 14, 17, 25, 33,
    38, 39, 49, 74, 95, 102–3,
    139, 163
sweet tastes 65, 142, 146
swimming 108, 157
swing phase 27

T

tactics and strategies 44, 46,
    59
target times 92, 114–15
technology, running 68–9
temperature, core *see* core/
    body temperature
tempo running 99
tendons *see* muscles,
    ligaments and tendons
thermoregulation 74–5,
    130
time zones, crossing 77
toe nails, losing 145–6, 152
Tokyo Marathon, Japan 159
topography, race 46
tops, running 49
training 18, 31, 50, 51, 57
altitude 71
boredom 83
breathing 67
calendar 180–1
cross-training 108–9
different approaches 88–9
final weeks and tapering
    122–4
friends/running clubs 80, 83,
    90, 91
importance of the 'long run'
    88–9, 95
interval 59, 62, 98–9
listen to your body 112
marginal gains 59

overtraining 118–20
pace 114–15
principles 82–4
programmes 84, 88, 90–1,
    96–7, 176–9
progression 59
schedules 31, 61, 88
specificity 58, 108
speed work 60, 62
starting out 80–1
time of day 76–7
treadmills 68
varying intensity 98–9
weekly mileage 62
treadmills, indoor 68, 87
triathlons and duathlons
    156–7

U

ultra-marathons 156, 162,
    164
urine colour 73, 103, 124,
    138
urine production 33, 138

V

visualisation 34, 65, 83
VO2 (volume of oxygen)
    20–1
VO2 max 21, 50, 62

W

walking 65, 147
warming down 22, 23, 72,
    104–5
warming up 22–3, 104
warmth, post-race 151
weather conditions 12, 39,
    46, 74–5, 106–7, 130–1,
    138, 140
weight gain 83, 125
weight loss 37, 39, 72–3, 95

ACKNOWLEDGEMENTS

With grateful thanks to Matt Lowing for his confidence in this book, and for his constant support and advice, and to Sarah Skipper for her editorial expertise and comments. Thanks to Beth Brewer for her proof reading and grammatical corrections, and thanks to Caroline, Emma and Beth for putting up with a runner who is always going to run "just one more marathon".

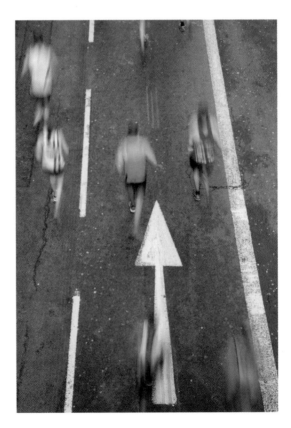